THE
GOOD
MOOD
DIET

THE
GOOD
MOOD
DIET

Feel Great While You Lose Weight

Susan M. Kleiner, PhD
with Bob Condor

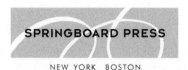

SPRINGBOARD PRESS

NEW YORK BOSTON

Springboard Press
Hachette Book Group USA
1271 Avenue of the Americas, New York, NY 10020
Visit our Web site at www.HachetteBookGroupUSA.com

Springboard Press is an imprint of Warner Books, Inc. The Springboard name and logo are trademarks of Hachette Book Group USA.

First Edition: January 2007

This book is intended as a reference volume only, not as a medical manual. The information provided is designed to help you make informed decisions about your health. It is not intended as a substitute for any treatment that may have been prescribed by your doctor. If you suspect that you have a medical problem, we urge you to seek competent medical help.

Library of Congress Cataloging-in-Publication Data
Kleiner, Susan M.
    The Good Mood Diet : feel great while you lose weight / by Susan M. Kleiner, with Bob Condor. — 1st ed.
        p. cm.
    Includes bibliographical references.
    ISBN-13: 978-0-8212-8004-1
    ISBN-10: 0-8212-8004-X
    1. Reducing diets — Popular works.   2. Weight loss — Popular works.
3. Food habits — Popular works.   4. Reducing diets — Recipes.
I. Condor, Bob.   II. Title.
RM222.2.K5655 2007
613.2'5 — dc22   2006015283

10 9 8 7 6 5 4 3 2 1

Printed in the United States of America

To Jeff, Danielle, and Ilana,
with joy in my heart.
— SMK

For Mary, Lana, and Arthur.
Then, now, always.
— BC

CONTENTS

THE
GOOD MOOD DIET

INTRODUCTION: FEEL GREAT WHILE YOU LOSE WEIGHT

I t's a funny thing for an author to say on the first page of her book, but I want you to stop reading for a moment after I ask this question: How are you feeling right now? Yes, I mean it. Stop. Think about the question.

How are you feeling?

Take a moment. Give yourself a body scan. And a mood check. How did you feel when you woke up this morning? What about yesterday? Do you ever know how you feel?

If you're like most people, you probably don't pay much attention to how you feel. A busy, demanding life has a way of doing that to even the most well-intentioned person. Tired . . . you go to work anyway. In pain . . . work through it. Hungry . . . grab something, even if it is junk or doesn't taste all that great. Sad . . . eat comfort foods, maybe talk to your doctor about a prescription antidepressant. Happy . . . fleeting, but we enjoy those moods when we can.

Well, there is one Big Fat Exception, like a movie that keeps playing over and over in our heads. We know exactly when we feel fat, which can be most of the time. What do we do when we feel fat? Go on a diet. It typically doesn't matter how bad it makes you feel, as long as you lose weight. Right?

Wrong. This book is all about explaining my answer. I will show you how to feel great while you lose weight. I will show you how your meals and snacks can put you in a good mood — every time.

The reason the Good Mood Diet works is because you will feel better on the diet. You will feel great. Your mood will lift, your energy will soar off the charts, and you won't feel hungry or cranky because you are missing out on foods you love.

The truth is, you won't even believe you are on a diet. Many of my clients find they have to get adjusted to eating more food, not less.

I will tell you about success stories and personal breakthroughs to make the Good Mood Diet come alive — and show how it fits into real life. I have worked directly with hundreds of people during my career as a nutritionist. They have come from all walks of life, ranging from a Super Bowl quarterback, to busy professionals and parents, to my own mother. Let's start with Jennifer Lail.

When I met Jennifer, she was upfront about feeling down and highly self-critical about herself — something lots of us might be less than willing to admit. She says she shook off a lifetime of self-doubt after just days on the Good Mood Diet.

"I'm thirty-five and always have been pretty healthy and active," says Jennifer, a Seattle woman who is involved in the sustainable housing industry. "But most of my life I've been plagued by body image hang-ups. Now I never think about them. My self-criticism and negativity just flipped to the positive."

Jennifer was among a group of *Seattle Post-Intelligencer* newspaper readers who agreed to engage in the highly public act of going on my Good Mood Diet. She lost 10 pounds and one clothing size in twelve weeks, reaching her initial goal. Five additional *Post-Intelligencer* readers lost 63 pounds total in the first three months, more than halfway to their personal long-term goals.

Better yet for Jennifer, she stopped having to "combat a consistent depression." Her depressive symptoms vanished with the Good Mood plan. Completely disappeared.

In one week.

"I used to get on my commuter ferry at night absolutely starved and grumpy," says Jennifer, who admits having tried many diets but never sticking to any one until she tried the Good Mood plan. "Now I am happy to wait for dinner."

Jennifer reaped almost instant benefits from the Good Mood plan. She saw rays of hope after just **one day** with a different food pattern and with sounder rest. In less than **one week** she no longer felt depressed. After **one month,** she lost 6 pounds and she does not anticipate gaining those extra pounds back. Why? Because she says she can "lose weight and feel normal" with the Good Mood Diet.

To prove the point: Jennifer lost 25 pounds during her first year of Good Mood eating and living.

"I love good food, and the amazing thing about this plan is that I honestly never feel hungry in a way that can't be satisfied with a Good Mood snack or meal," says Jennifer. "It is second nature now to grab for something that supports health rather than something that detracts from it."

Jennifer pauses and smiles. "Plus," she adds, "I can still have a glass of wine with friends."

Jennifer's experience is a familiar pattern to me. I have lost count of how many times a client or newspaper reader has called or emailed to remark how "great" they feel or "how much more energy I have for work or my family."

I will be "keeping it real" throughout this book with ways to fit this diet into your life — and not the other way around. For example, the fourteen days of Good Mood Menus in Chapter 3 all come with Real Life notes that cover such issues as the best time to have a smoothie, eating lunch out, or fitting pizza into the plan.

And, yes, that includes chocolate.

Let's talk real life. When I talked about the Good Mood Diet to a group of about 350 people in Cleveland, there was some concern about my recommendation to eat five fish meals each week, preferably a cold-water fish such as salmon or tuna. People were concerned about finding fresh fish, at least in some seasons, plus the cost. We'll talk more about why salmon and tuna are such stellar mood and brain foods, but here's my real-life answer to those questioners in Cleveland: Five fish meals a week is your goal — and I have plenty of ideas about how to add canned tuna and salmon to your meals without high expense — but if you eat, say, only two or three, that's still two or three times a week you have boosted your mood with omega-3 fats.

Or maybe you have catfish or walleye instead of wild salmon or low-mercury tuna (much more about this in Chapter 1); that's still a healthy measure more of omega-3 fats than you would get from a hamburger or pork roast. But, hey, real life wins out sometimes, hamburgers and pork roast can be part of the Good Mood Diet too. Pork, especially, is bursting with B vitamins that control stress, and the neurotransmitter choline that helps fuel the brain.

This revolutionary Good Mood regime is developed from my twenty-five years of professional experience as a nutritionist. I have worked with professional sports teams, advised top-flight business executives and, oh, about a thousand mothers with young kids and their husbands looking to stave off middle age.

Feel brighter today than yesterday.

Why the Good Mood Diet? Because we can all use a lift in our mood and fill-up for the energy tank. It's more lasting than even weight loss. On restrictive diets, people can lose pounds but also lose steam. The Good Mood Plan is one you can live with — happily — for a lifetime. It is about the food you *need* to eat, not about food you can't eat.

"Like most people, I thought that in order to lose weight, you had to drastically reduce calories," says Sherry Bencetic, a forty-four-year-old client who lives in Pittsburgh. "But the Good Mood Diet showed me why you can't get the desired results if you don't eat the proper amount of calories to fuel your body."

What excites me is people who quickly refocus from losing weight to gaining a "Wow" perspective about their energy and vibrancy. They tell me, "I feel terrific, I feel so much more awake and alive, and, oh yeah, I lost eight pounds."

Most diets, unfortunately, cause chemical changes in the brain that make the dieter feel depressed. The typical plan is most often too low in calories (repeat after me: too low in calories) to fuel a day's worth of energy for a small pigeon — much less for an active adult.

Here's a big and important difference in the Good Mood Diet plan: Participants eat what I call Feel-Great Foods with both ideal timing and in ideal combinations. During waking hours, you will consume a meal or snack every two to three hours. Even before bedtime, you drink a hot cocoa to encourage sleep and satisfy any lingering appetite. Many clients and readers report that this bedtime cup of cocoa becomes a soothing ritual that is shared with their spouses.

Strange thing, many of my clients who start the plan say their challenge is to eat enough food throughout the day. See if this sounds familiar: The typical American adult is accustomed to skipping breakfast, keeping busy through lunch or choosing low-fat options (such as the dreaded and dreary green salad with low-fat dressing and nothing else on the table), then feeling starved at dinner. That's a recipe for eating too much at the wrong times. The Good Mood plan encourages you never to feel hungry — and that keeps your emotions positively fueled all day.

Your energy levels will soar in days. This is not a hollow promise. You will feel so much better in just days. Guaranteed.

It's all about how you feel.

Why do you have to feel so lousy, so deprived, so depressed when you are on a diet? I say it's possible to feel great while you lose weight.

Make that *really* great.

"My energy has been great," says Felicity Mansanarez, a thirty-one-year-old nurse, after less than one month on the Good Mood program. "And it seems, strangely enough, that I have more patience."

Felicity changed employers during her first weeks on the Good Mood Diet. She adjusted without a problem to starting hospital work at 6:00 a.m. three days a week. The other mornings, she still gets up early to follow a home video aerobic weight training circuit or attend kickboxing class.

"I feel stronger and my back, usually a weak spot, hasn't given me any trouble at all," she says.

During her first year on the Good Mood plan, Felicity fell in love. She was engaged just thirteen months after starting the diet. Now, in that area, I make no guarantees. But, seriously, Felicity is the first to acknowledge she is happier than she's ever been. "The biggest benefit that I've found with this diet is energy," she says. "My stress level is down considerably, or maybe I should say my ability to deal with stress has improved. I've benefited from both the diet and the increased exercise that the eating plan helps me to sustain. I plan to continue the eating program, no doubt."

Let me say a few words about exercise here. I am a believer that no one loses weight and, more important, keeps off the pounds, without being physically active. When someone asks me what percentage of losing weight is diet and what percentage is exercise, I am tempted to say 50/50 or something like that to get optimal results. But, honestly, the answer is 100/100. You will succeed to the highest degree when you give a 100 percent in both areas.

The Good Mood Diet is not an all-or-nothing plan.

Any changes you make, such as adding a cup of hot cocoa to your bedtime routine or always combining protein, carbs, and healthy fats in every snack, will boost your mood and feed your brain. You will feel the difference and, as happens with nearly every one of my clients, you will start looking for more ways to stay in the Good Mood groove. That's an important point and is especially valuable to remember when life gets stressful.

For starters, I recommend exercise that literally fits into your life by setting a Good Mood goal of taking 10,000 steps per day.

A pedometer does the counting, something that will be discussed in Chapter 6. The typical American takes about 6,000 steps per day, so I am only asking for 4,000 more in many cases. Even the most sedentary individuals take about 3,000 daily steps. If you reach the 10,000-step goal most days, it will directly impact how much weight you lose — and keep off. Invest in a good-quality pedometer.

You will feel more rested, no small accomplishment.

Sleep and rest don't get much attention in diet books. I will make the argument that research shows not getting enough sleep actually will sabotage your weight-loss goals. Here's why: Your body goes into survival mode when it doesn't get enough rest, a leftover effect from our prehistoric caveman roots. The brain and body assume there is some sort of pending danger or strife. And all because you wanted to watch that late-night movie on cable.

During his first three months on the Good Mood plan as part of the *Seattle Post-Intelligencer* trial group, Patrick D'Amelio noticed some distinct patterns. For instance, he found he handled stress better. He didn't feel deprived and "never felt starved." His energy level zoomed.

Plus, Patrick lost 35 pounds in three months.

"People at work, family and friends, they all noticed the weight loss," says Patrick, who is the chief executive officer of Big Brothers Big Sisters of Seattle and Tacoma. "But they also noticed I just look better — more rested and healthier."

Patrick's newfound energy affords him, by his estimate, an extra hour or two every day. "I wake up refreshed, and an hour or two before the alarm," he says.

Practically all of my clients report the same thing. What I typically hear within one week is, "I have so much more energy."

Moreover, my clients who are parents with young kids discover the stamina to actually stay awake to talk with their spouses after the kids go to bed. In fact, a good number of mothers have tailored their Good Mood plan for the whole family. Kids eat healthier, there are fewer household arguments and, get this, temper tantrums disappear about as fast as the depression is lifted. One of my clients, whose son routinely embarrassed her with public tantrums, said his outbursts completely stopped after about a month on a modified Good Mood plan.

What's wrong with other diets is that most all of them cause chemical changes in your brain that make you feel depressed.

The typical weight-loss plan is simply too low in calories to fuel a day's worth of energy for an adult looking to lead a quality life. It's a prescription for feeling just how you don't want to feel: lousy, no energy, and craving foods that will give you instant gratification and naturally elevate your mood. Yet you can't have those foods you crave — including fallen-from-favor carbs. You can't eat the foods that will boost your mood and make your day. Figure that!

Note to breakfast cereal lovers: You will be delighted to know that cereal can be a regular part of a Good Mood breakfast — or even substitute as a snack. I talk to clients and Web visitors (www.goodmooddiet.com) every week who are excited about bringing cold cereal back into their mornings.

Personally, I am a shredded wheat fan from way back. I also love the Kashi line of cold cereals. But feel free to roam the cereal aisle at the store (we take an extended grocery store tour in Chapter 4). There is an impressive selection of whole-grain, fiber-rich cereals that taste just as good, I swear and so do many clients, as the cereals we all munched on as kids.

Always combine carbs, protein, and fat.

A key Good Mood strategy is to combine your *macronutrients*. For instance, a mid-afternoon apple snack needs a balance of protein and fats (nut butter is one example, or nuts, or a low-fat cheese stick) to go with the carbs in the apple. Our brain and muscles actually crave the protein powder in a mid-morning smoothie — or the protein in an egg-white omelet — then use that protein to stay more even-keeled.

My clients always make sure they are never eating only carbs. For example, adding ground flaxseed to a morning meal boosts mood virtually instantly. Healthy fats are good fats. Adding olive oil to a midday salad or as part of a turkey sandwich will work wonders in a participant's overall emotional state.

Sherry Bencetic, my client in Pittsburgh, credits this food combining with helping her lose the extra weight she couldn't trim for years. She lost 8 pounds in eight weeks, and dropped her body fat percentage from 24.5 to 20 percent in that time. "I'm one of those women who struggled for years to lose the 'last ten pounds,' " she says. "I hired a personal trainer and I tried every kind of diet, but to no avail. The Good Mood plan taught me the importance of eating the right combinations of foods at the right time of the day. I'm convinced that's how I finally lost the weight."

A Good Mood Breakthrough Story:

A MOTHER LODE APPROACH

A great test case for the Seattle Good Mood Diet comes right from my own eighty-four-year-old mother. Mom has always been a happy, enthusiastic person. My dad passed away eleven years ago, and as often happens in these situations, she became mildly depressed (and gained a few pounds). But she slowly came out of it.

Then one day Mom seemed unusually blue for someone who always put on a happy face. It just wasn't like her at all.

Tapping into my experience as a nutritionist, I suggested she make fresh salmon or halibut (rub with oil and broil it) four or five days a week. I urged her to add flax meal to her cereal and eat a whole egg (the yolk is a brain- and mood-enhancer) every day.

We also talked about getting sunlight every day for fifteen minutes, taking a vitamin D supplement during the darker winter months, and trying to avoid the added sugar in processed foods (including cereals and sweets and even checking the labels for sugar content in yogurt).

And it all worked. Mom felt better about herself within days. She shed the extra pounds she'd gained over nine years. She loved the meals she could now prepare without guilt. It all added up to a Good Mood Breakthrough of the most personal and happy kind for me.

Mood is the huge missing link in weight-loss strategies.

No matter what the goals of my clients, I always keep mood in mind. It is simply overlooked in most every other diet. For instance, people who have tried high-protein diets lose major pounds in the early weeks or months, but over the longer term they become mean and crabby. So they go off the diet and gain all the weight back again, and more. So I am decidedly against zero- or low-carb meals and snacks but still endorse significant intakes of lean protein (about 30 percent of daily calories).

My clients and Good Mood Diet followers eat about 40 percent carbs and roughly 30 percent fats. The carbs are healthy varieties, mostly fruits, vegetables, and whole grains rather than any processed foods with added sugar. The elimination of added sugar in processed foods is a cornerstone strategy for both mood and weight.

In the Good Mood Diet, sweets are not taboo. But I advise an eat-it-only-if-you-love-it approach. If you love pumpkin pie, have a slice — but maybe skip the crust unless it is fabulous.

Even Super Bowl quarterbacks have a sweet tooth.

When I first worked with Super Bowl star Matt Hasselbeck, the Seattle Seahawks quarterback, he was eating at least a pint of ice cream every night and was kidded by his teammates for eating four, sometimes even five, Dove bars on a return flight from an away game. Matt wasn't fighting any weight problems, but he wasn't feeling totally sharp. In fact, his goal was to gain muscle weight.

Matt and I drew up an eating game plan that still allowed him a generous portion of ice cream at night. After a little more than a week, Matt called with a report and a request. "I feel so good," he told me. "I don't even crave the ice cream anymore. What other healthier snacks can I eat at bedtime?"

The Good Mood Diet will work for you.

There are several integral reasons why the Good Mood Diet and this book will help you meet elusive weight-loss goals, plus help you feel great and stay that way. If performing better at work or sports is your goal, the Good Mood Diet will achieve those goals too. Same goes for improving the relationships in your life and finding the energy to chase your dreams. Here's why I guarantee you will prosper with the Good Mood Plan:

The Good Mood Diet offers the most powerful motivator:
Feeling great while you lose weight.

Weight loss is a great motivator to start a diet, but it's not enough to sustain you through the tough times. How you feel is much more powerful. Most weight-loss diets are inherently depressing. So you go on them, follow them diligently, feel lousy, and then go off the diet. Then you regain all the weight and feel lousy again. Feeling good is part of the Good Mood plan. If you feel good, you keep following the plan, and if you need to lose weight, you will.

The Good Mood Diet operates from a science-based assumption:
There are Feel-Great Foods and Feel-Bad Foods.

We will talk about Feel-Great Foods in Chapter 1 and Feel-Bad Foods in Chapter 2, but to start, here are some of the most powerful Feel-Great Foods: turkey, milk, cocoa powder, eggs, fish, coffee (1 to 2 cups before noon), lean pork, blueberries, air-popped popcorn, oranges, olive oil, and sunflower seeds.

The Feel-Bad Foods are the foods that often give us immediate gratification in the pleasure category, but make us feel lousy in the long run. It's a short list that includes alcohol (can move to the Feel-Great category when consumed in moderation), caffeine in large doses, fried foods, fatty meats, fatty snack foods, added sugar.

The first two weeks of the Good Mood Diet have such a powerful impact on mood that you won't ever want to go back to the way you felt before.

The first two weeks of the plan eliminate the Feel-Bad Foods and provide bountiful Feel-Great choices. The menu plans are based on the typical calorie needs for women and men of different sizes and activity levels: 1,600 or 1,800 or 2,200 calories, all fully explained in Chapter 3. There is a two-week abstinence from alcohol that troubles some Good Mood Dieters at first but quickly becomes a positive in the program. For instance, people learn greater body awareness, how alcohol can cloud relationships, and even that less alcohol significantly lowers the grocery bill.

Your reward for those first two weeks? Dark chocolate and red wine become part of your plan.

"I came to realize that I was gobbling chocolate chip cookies to stuff down the stress in my life," says Paula Burke, a business consultant with two toddlers at home. "Now I really savor a good piece of chocolate, taking the time to take pleasure in it."

You don't have to be perfect or even close to it.

Eating Good Mood foods is the key strategy of the Good Mood Diet, not avoiding foods. Even if you "slip" in your goals, make sure you include Feel-Great Foods at every meal and snack to brighten your mood. Plus, oh, how great is this, you will lose weight naturally while adding red wine and chocolate back to your day.

It's not about eliminating foods you love, but about appreciating them more.

1

FEEL-GREAT FOODS

Here is a switch in eating that you will no doubt savor. The Good Mood plan emphasizes what foods to eat each day, not what foods to avoid. Those foods you want to eat are what I call Feel-Great Foods. They will change your whole attitude from "can't have" to "can do."

Just ask Patrick D'Amelio, the forty-year-old chief executive officer of Big Brothers Big Sisters in Seattle and Tacoma. Patrick is an accomplished fund-raiser and highly visible community member. People by the hundreds look up to him as a leader.

But in his personal life, Patrick struggled. He was some 60 pounds overweight and just not feeling 100 percent physically, mentally, even spiritually. He feared his years of yo-yo dieting and crash workout programs were catching up with him.

Patrick discovered my list of Feel-Great Foods. He was thrilled to learn that my Good Mood plan emphasized what foods to eat each day — not what foods to avoid or, worse yet, feel guilty about splurging on or straying off the plan.

Within the first week, Patrick said his energy level shot upward. After one month, he'd lost 16 pounds, then 35 pounds in his first three Good

Mood months. Best of all, he dropped the weight almost without thinking about it. All he did was select from the list of Feel-Great Foods (see below) for most of his meal and snack choices. He quickly memorized his favorites, including nuts of all kinds, part-skim mozzarella string cheese, and, wow, burgers.

The Good Mood Diet is all about choosing Feel-Great Foods — without guilt.

My eating plan is the kinder, gentler approach to taking care of you. No more self-abuse through deprivation. No more days with so little energy that you can't get out of bed. No more days where you feel so mean that you hurt the people you love or ignore the coworkers who are most critical to your job success. And best of all, the Good Mood Diet means no more guilt.

Feel-Great Foods give back your favorite meals and snacks. You can eat breakfast cereal (skip the sugar-coated) after years of carbohydrate-guilt. You can eat an egg a day, drink a strong cup of coffee in the morning, have a bowl of chili for lunch, eat nuts and string cheese at snack time, and order tacos or steak or a pork chop for dinner.

Every client that I work with gets a diet plan designed with goals of both feeling great and losing weight/body fat built into it. Not a week goes by that I don't hear from a client who says the nutrition program has changed his or her life. Even the most naturally exuberant of my clients claim that they feel better than ever, within days.

The list of Feel-Great Foods is your starter kit for wiping away the guilt. It works hand-in-hand with the menus in Chapter 3 to give you a food plan and lifetime philosophy. Simply, you eat to feel good. The weight loss will take care of itself. Here's the list. It highlights the optimal foods that should be part of your daily diet as spelled out in Chapter 3. Of course, there are other Feel-Great Food categories, such as pretty much all fruits and vegetables. What this list does — different from many diets — is identify the fresh produce (or flash-frozen) most able to boost your mood.

FEEL-GREAT FOODS

Bananas	Greens, dark and leafy
Beans	Green tea
Blueberries	Lean, organic meat
Broccoli	Mangoes
Caffeine-containing beverages	Nuts
(1 to 2 each day)	Olives and olive oil
Cocoa powder (or chocolate in	Oranges
small amounts)	Pomegranates
Dairy, low-fat or fat-free	Popcorn, air-popped
Edamame (green soybeans)	Pork, lean
Egg yolks	Soy
Fish and seafood	Spinach
Flaxseed, ground	Strawberries
Garlic	Sunflower seeds
Ginger	Turkey, light and dark meat
Grapefruit	Vegetable oil, unrefined
Grape juice	Whole grains

I have developed this list of Feel-Great Foods from years of working with elite athletes, businesspeople, mothers with young kids, and all types of other clients. There is good science to prove its effectiveness, and even better real-life trial and error evidence.

Here's one example: Several years ago I worked with an all-star NBA player who had fallen into a depression. It didn't matter how fit he was, he couldn't perform on the court. It was my job not only to get him back into playing shape, but to give him back his mental focus. I designed his diet with both of these goals in mind, drawing liberally from the Feel-Great list.

The results were amazing. In five weeks he lowered his body fat by 10 percent. This required not only following the diet, but having the mental energy, focus, exuberance, and physical energy to return to his usual activities and training, with a drive to win.

There's no place for guilt on this diet. Even if you eat something that's not on the Feel-Great Foods list, you still need to eat all the rest of the foods planned for the day. Don't tweak the diet to make up for the calories. I don't care if you ate half of a chocolate cake five minutes ago; I still want you to eat all the foods that are on the plan that make you feel great. As long as you keep feeling great, you'll avoid eating the other half of the cake. The guilt will just drive you to eat more cake. Let it go.

This is the eating plan to end your diet misery.

Have you ever been on a diet? Of course you have. You've followed it diligently, only to fall off after a few months (or even a few weeks or days) with a loud thud.

Why did you stop? You felt lousy, had no energy, your cravings went out of control — and that was the end. You droop your shoulders and fret about another failure of your body and your willpower.

But wait. Upon closer examination, you now should realize the flaw was with the diet you were following, not with you. Rather than continuing to think that everything is wrong with you and your body, it could be that the diet doesn't hold together.

The fact is most diets are inherently depressing. The way these diets are put together and the foods they dictate you should eat cause chemical changes in your brain that actually make you feel depressed. The problem is obvious in some ways but commonly overlooked: Most diets are much too low in calories. Not only will you feel sluggish and, well, moody in all of the wrong ways, you are denying yourself foods that give you instant fuel and provide the pick-me-up we all crave, especially during the day.

Oh, and did I mention lousy?

You may initially have lost weight quickly on a fad diet and been happy, even elated, with the results. But over time, your desire to lose weight lessened and even disappeared. You could barely get through the day without feeling you would rather be somebody else, anybody who could order a bagel with a smear or tacos or a lamb chop without feeling like you were cheating. The only person you were cheating was yourself.

The Good Mood Diet lets you be yourself — and lets you pick your own favorite Feel-Great Foods to fuel your upbeat moods and chase away depressive symptoms.

One example for egg lovers: All of the negative press about eggs is messing with one of the best foods for your brain and your temperament.[1] I recommend that you eat one whole egg per day (the yolk contains lecithin, which works wonders for brain cells) — especially in the morning, if possible.

If your cardiologist recommends against a daily egg and makes a reasonable case for why it compromises your cholesterol levels and heart disease risk, ask how many yolks per week is acceptable to boost brainpower without compromising your cardio health. On days when you don't eat a yolk, substitute a whole soy food like tofu or edamame (buy them frozen still in the pod, steam them and lightly salt for a satisfying snack or even a breakfast side dish). The benefits are found in the fat part of soy, so soy protein alone won't substitute for the egg.

And don't neglect egg whites. The protein in whites is superb for muscle building, and a four-egg-white omelet (with a side glass of fat-free milk) can substitute for the Good Mood Diet mid-morning smoothie that is a staple of the menus in Chapter 3.

Prepare your whole egg any way you like, even as part of a Good Mood pancake recipe. Eating foods with some fat, like egg yolk, helps us feel more satisfied after meals. Forget fat-phobia. The fear of fat can actually make you fatter and certainly grumpier. That's why the Good Mood snack lineup features fat-containing almonds and other nuts.

Try this on your next sandwich: Use your favorite condiments but add a teaspoon of olive oil. You will feel more satisfied the hour or two after the sandwich — and you'll get a burst of energy that seems to come out of nowhere but is directly from the healthy monounsaturated fats in the olive oil.

What may have gone wrong with your other diets is that you either got no fat, healthy or unhealthy, or that you feasted on fatty animal foods. I still find it hard to grasp how much bacon some people have consumed on high-protein, low-carb diets.

Here's why both the no-fat or high-fat diets may have crashed on you. Your body's natural defense mechanisms kicked in to prevent disaster. While you may assume that losing weight required a painful, uncomfortable process, your body knows better.

When such a process throws you off track — way off track in most cases — your body responds with a survival tactic established millennia ago. It makes it nearly impossible to lose any more weight.

Starving yourself doesn't drop pounds, but likely will do just the opposite.

In fact, deprivation diets do accomplish just the opposite. Your body braces itself to *not* lose weight.

One result is that you feel lethargic and, well, moody in all the wrong ways. You are impelled to eat high-fat, high-sugar foods to ward off the blues. You crave a different way of living, and reaching for cookies or chips is a natural response.

Remember this, especially if a friend or loved one or counselor urges you to reach down deep for your willpower. You're not broken, your diet is, and your body is working as it is meant to, protecting you from the damage that can come from an inadequate diet.

Forget that whole no-willpower guilt trip. Not to sound sappy, but we have one life here, guys. Nobody says you have to live it starving all the time to demonstrate to the world that you have a strong will. Fuel your body and mind with the Good Mood plan, and your will and your happiness will follow.

The Good Mood Diet is both a food plan and a lifetime philosophy. I want you to think like the athletes that I've worked with for twenty-five years do. They are tremendously optimistic. All they think about is doing what they *need* to do to be successful. They follow a plan for success. If they step off the path, most just get right back on again and keep following their plan. Food is their fuel, their friend; not their enemy. They don't waste time thinking about what doesn't work, or what they didn't do right. Their focus is on doing what it takes to be, and stay, in top form.

On a daily basis, I want you to think about what you *need* to eat, not what you can't eat. You must feed your brain to feel great. What's more, the care and feeding of your brain in the Good Mood Diet will recalibrate your ability to burn fat and build muscle after years or maybe decades of a yo-yo metabolism. You will be leaner but not meaner.

Your brain is the control center. The brain allows the release of neuro-transmitters and hormones that change your body from a fat-making machine into a fat-burning machine. Until your brain is in nutritional balance, the switch will never happen.

That's why even when you think you're doing everything right, you don't lose weight. You have to feed your brain first. That's the initial step you need to feel great.

Imagine that. The first step to losing weight is to make sure you are feeling great. That is a happy difference in my plan. If you feel great, then you stick with it. And if you stick with the plan, you lose weight. It's that simple. Cause and effect is a powerful tool for self-enhancement.

Bottom line, weight loss should be exhilarating. But on most diets it's depressing. That's because the nature of the diet plan actually makes you depressed. Not so with the Good Mood Diet. Remember my credo: Feel great while you lose weight.

Thinking about what you need to eat starts at breakfast.

The Feel-Great list is nearly as long as it is comforting. For many Good Mood Dieters with whom I've worked, the wide choice of breakfast items is a big plus. People love the idea of toast, eggs, cold cereal, oatmeal, yogurt, English muffin egg sandwiches, sausages, and even French toast. My own a.m. favorites include bite-size shredded wheat (I know, boring, but it works for me). I eat it with fat-free milk when I first wake up, which is usually about an hour before our children are up. Then I eat an egg and some fruit with my children during their breakfast.

I save my morning coffee to drink while sitting with the kids, too, but lots of my clients prefer the caffeine first thing. That fits into the Good Mood plan, no problem. In fact, unlike many diets, my plan advocates that a cup or two of coffee (or one to two shots of espresso) is ideal for most people, especially devoted coffee drinkers. Research is clear that caffeine enhances physical and mental performance in moderate amounts.[2]

What's more, a morning latte is truly both a Feel-Great drink and a treat. I suggest espresso drinks because you can be sure of not overdoing it. Yet I trust you to figure out how much caffeine is just right and how much turns to jitters or nervousness or that jumpy-mind feeling any coffee drinker recognizes. For the record, if a client insists on an ounce count, I mark out a "tall cup" or 12 ounces of strongly brewed coffee as the day's ideal amount. That can reach to 16 ounces for some individuals or drop to 8 to 10 for the more coffee-sensitive.

In any case, my Good Mood plan strongly suggests drinking the coffee before lunch, then switching to green tea or water for afternoon breaktime beverages. You can figure on up to three additional cups of green tea, or five total if you prefer it over coffee. I'm a big fan of green tea for its gentle mood pick-me-up and its abundance of antioxidants and other cancer and heart disease protectors.

Just to show you how much feel-great range the Good Mood plan offers, I am even OK with a diet cola or two in the mornings if that is your caffeine drink of choice. Just skip the "regular" versions (the typical 12-ounce can has 10 teaspoons of added sugar) and bust your afternoon and evening soft drink habits to boost mood and energy.

Try a week without soft drinks if you don't believe me. You will feel better simply by substituting water or green tea for post-noon sodas. If you are a carbonated drink fan, then try easing into the new pattern by pouring yourself a sparkling water over ice with a splash of your favorite fruit juice.

Increasing how much food you eat during the day means less weight gain and calmer nerves — even for young kids.

Sharon Lee Hamilton is a forty-nine-year-old mother with two young children. She loves the Good Mood diet for how it limits the effects of stress in her life.

"I felt more calm around the kids, and last year we went through some challenging times during a foreign adoption process," says Sharon. "Rather than gain weight during all that, which is what normally happens, I lost four pounds."

One of Sharon's successful strategies was making sure to eat a Good

Mood breakfast every day. She experimented with the Good Mood Menus (Chapter 3) and recipes (Chapter 8) to find dishes that worked for her busy life. One of her favorites was an English-muffin egg sandwich with olive oil rather than cheese. Another was a hard-boiled egg and a yogurt fruit parfait that she would make the night before for a fast exit from the house.

"I just loved eating a meal in the morning, yet it only takes me minutes to get everything ready, even if I toast the muffin and cook the egg," says Sharon. "Grabbing a healthy breakfast, heck, just eating breakfast, has made a huge difference for me. Plus, I see the same benefits in getting breakfast into my young children."

Bingo on that one. How many parents do you know who believe in feeding their children a healthy, fortifying breakfast, but only drink coffee because they are "not morning eaters." That's what I call a Feel-Bad strategy. Picking some Feel-Great Foods, even if they are traditional breakfast foods, will pay dividends.

A number of my clients make a smoothie for breakfast to save on time and help make the mental adjustment to eating in the morning. I highly recommend my Eye-Opener Smoothie made with milk and chai tea (see next page).

Good Mood smoothie recipes (see Chapter 8) can also help you persuade your teenagers to follow a healthier morning food routine. With teens, I find it is more successful to discuss improving mood rather than body weight. I have worked with a good number of teens and youth programs. This age group responds to a focus on power and personal energy. Teens are bombarded with messages about body image; I want them thinking about feeling better and more hopeful. The Good Mood Diet fits the bill.

Plus, smoothies are a good breakfast or mid-morning option for teens who sleep until the last minute (sound familiar?). And you might know the research, but it is documented by sleep scientists that adolescents do indeed have a harder time falling asleep at night due to hormonal differences than either younger children or adults. The right type of smoothie can get them back in balance.

Eye-Opener Smoothie

1 cup fat-free milk
1 Chai tea bag
14 grams protein from vanilla isolated whey protein powder
1 teaspoon Splenda
⅛ teaspoon nutmeg
4 ice cubes

Heat the milk in the microwave and pour over the tea bag; steep 5 to 8 minutes. Discard the tea bag. Cool the milk in the refrigerator for 20 minutes or even overnight. Pour the milk into a blender and add the protein powder, Splenda, nutmeg, and ice cubes. Blend 1 minute, until smooth.

Makes 1 serving.

Good Mood analysis:

Each serving contains 1 milk; 2 very lean proteins

A few words about the whey protein: I recommend isolated whey protein because it allows you to control your protein for peak brain and body benefits. Some protein powders and whey powders contain carbs and even fats that you don't want or need for the best mood lift. This shake is particularly valuable right after exercise but also works wonders for many of my clients as a mid-morning snack no matter when they exercise.

Eating fish is a strategic step to eliminating depression but doesn't have to break your budget.

For some of us — I'm raising my hand — eating salmon three to five times each week is a major plus in the Good Mood plan. While fresh salmon can get pricey in some regions — look for sales and freeze individual portions — you don't need more than 4 ounces for the mood boost.

In fact, I can make a strong argument that eating salmon and other oily, cold-water fish is a sure antidote to depression symptoms. It certainly worked that way for my own mother (see Good Mood Breakthrough, page 9). It is almost too simple for some people to accept that the omega-3 fats in fish curb depression, but I see it firsthand with dozens of clients every year.

An alternative to fresh fish is canned salmon. Try some different brands to figure out the tastier versions and what fits into your food budget. Keep a few cans in your pantry for quick-fix dinners that will serve your mood for hours and help you sleep better.

Though living in the Northwest, Patrick D'Amelio was not much of a fish eater. That challenged one of the Feel-Great food strategies, which promotes cold-water fish rich in omega-3 fats. Examples include salmon, tuna, sardines, and anchovies.

At our first meeting of the Seattle newspaper trial group, Patrick admitted he didn't really like salmon, which is sort of like a Chicagoan saying no thanks to deep-dish pizza. I countered that most people eat canned tuna, a budgetary bargain for its Good Mood quotient. Patrick agreed he could certainly fit tuna into his meals three to five times per week.

One problem: Commercial-brand canned tuna can be high in mercury content.[3] I talked to Patrick about trying troll-caught tuna, such as the Fishing Vessel St. Jude brand (www.tunatuna.com), because it tastes delicious, plus is much fresher and more appetizing than commercially caught tuna. Importantly, troll-caught tuna has no, or at most trace amounts of, mercury, primarily because troll fishing hooks smaller fish that haven't built up the mercury load big tuna get from eating other sizable fish and from simply living longer.

Another big plus is that troll-caught tuna keeps its omega-3 potency because the small-company fishermen and independent operators keep their fish intact. Large-scale commercial tuna fishing boats trim off most fat and oils at sea because Americans don't like the smell of fish. Problem is, deodorizing greatly reduces the healthy omega-3 fat content. The healthy amount is 7 grams of fat per serving, while some of the large-scale brands have as little as ½ to 1 gram. You pay less, but get way less.

"The low-mercury tuna costs more [roughly four dollars a can], but it is more than worth it," said Patrick after picking up some Fishing Vessel St. Jude. "It makes great sandwiches and burritos."

Yes, you're reading right. Burritos fit the Good Mood Diet. So do hamburgers, mashed potatoes, pork chops, pasta, and hot cocoa. This is a diet that doesn't make you die for something good to eat.

Not eating foods that make you feel great is not acceptable. It doesn't make sense. Food is to be enjoyed, life is to be lived — not spent lamenting all of the favorite meals you feel compelled to miss.

One more important point: Five fish meals a week is your goal, not an ultimatum or five-or-bust proposition. Every fish meal is a plus for the omega-3 fat content — and your brain.

One common goal for all of my clients is that nobody goes hungry.

Now I admit that we will be retraining your palate in this book, especially by adding some new staples to your meal plans (ground flaxseed, for instance). But this by no means has to be at the price of hunger pangs or the brightness of your psyche or both.

"I was never hungry, not once," says Patrick, looking back on his first twelve weeks, when he lost 35 pounds but notched even more meaningful changes. "It was almost like I was glowing. The weight loss was more like, 'oh, right, you lost weight too.' "

Another client who never felt hungry was Linda Behlke. She joined one of my Good Mood Diet Clubs that have formed since the diet was first publicized. For Linda, one of the best things about the Good Mood Diet is not feeling like she has to be perfect.

"It was clear from the start of our diet club, nobody is going to be perfect," says Linda. "Every other diet I have tried — and I have tried them all — you feel like either you do it perfectly or you are a failure."

Here's an important point about the Good Mood Diet. If you don't quite follow the Good Mood Menus some days, don't sweat it — but do your best to still eat the Good Mood foods such as one egg, your daily serving of ground flaxseed, the whey protein shake, and hot cocoa before bed. You will still be doing something positive even on the most stressful days.

Linda lost 12 pounds in her first three months of the Good Mood plan — and that was during the winter holidays season. She especially likes "shrinking" into clothes that were too small just weeks before.

"Things are going *great!*" says Linda. "I'm amazed that I don't have any cravings and it seems painless to follow the program — I'm not tempted to overeat or indulge."

Linda has a special reason to appreciate the Good Mood plan. She has multiple sclerosis. "It can cause major fatigue," Linda says. "With Dr. Kleiner's plan, I have so much more energy and hope."

And fewer pounds.

Weight a minute: There's much more to my plan than losing pounds.

Beyond the weight loss, the Good Mood Diet aims squarely at helping people gain more energy and feel good about themselves, both traits that my coauthor, Bob, writes about in his newspaper columns. We kept this in mind when creating a trial group for the *Post-Intelligencer.* Not everyone approached the diet with the primary goal of losing weight.

In fact, when Patrick D'Amelio first walked into the newspaper conference room with its sweeping view of Puget Sound, he had made a snap judgment.

"Oh, I'm in the wrong place," he thought to himself as he looked around at the folks gathering in the room. "These people don't need to lose any weight." But he quickly realized that one person's 60 pounds can be another person's 10 or 20. That was apparent from listening to others in the test group.

"I come from a family of Southern petite women," said Jennifer Lail, who would become a Good Mood devotee, losing twenty-five pounds and three clothing sizes in her first year on the plan. "But I guess I got my body from my father's side of the family. I like to call myself petite stocky."

Everyone in the room easily smiled at Jennifer's lines, but her comments just as suddenly caused each person to grow quiet. Jennifer was opening up, making the rest of us reflect on past hurts and shaky moments about our bodies. I hoped only that Jennifer would give the Good Mood Diet a fair chance. I knew my approach could change everything for her.

No worries there.

"The biggest compliment I get from people is when they ask me about getting more information about the Good Mood Diet," says Jennifer. "They tell me they are so impressed with not just how I look but how they feel around me. It's like my feeling better makes them feel better — and more hopeful."

You might wonder why I call it the Good Mood Diet. Here's the quick story line: I live in the Seattle area, where we sporadically get some of the world's greatest weather in the spring, summer, and fall. But the payback is having to endure wet, gray, and short days — dark until 8:30 a.m. and dark again by 4:00 p.m. — during November, December, January, and part of February.

I have found over the years that my eating plans for hundreds of clients have not only helped them lose weight, but have improved their moods dramatically. No more feeling blue or sluggish. The Good Mood Diet has helped local professional athletes perform better and — happily for fans — even convinced them to keep playing for their Seattle team rather than run off to a sunnier climate.

"You saved my life," one businesswoman client emailed after just ten days on the diet. "I am picking the right foods and I feel fantastic. I just never knew what foods could make me feel this good. I have more hope in my life."

For me, hope equals Good Mood. In the early days of the plan, you will feel instant boosts in your energy and ability to sleep. You will feel more alive, brighter-minded. The Good Mood continues on as you start to drop pounds and/or feel muscle taking over where flab has reigned. And for anyone who suffers even mild depression, the featured foods in this diet will act as servings of Good Mood.

I've lost count of the number of clients who report feeling depressed when we first meet, only to report happier and more hopeful days after just one week. Sometimes people can't wait a week for a positive report, emailing me or calling on their cell phone within the first twenty-four or forty-eight hours. It's almost as if the mid-morning smoothie or afternoon snack or bedtime cocoa is acting like an eraser on depression. People are rubbing it out day by day.

What a wonderful concept, connecting food with hope and energy and feeling good. That's why I call it the Good Mood Diet.

Welcome to the rest of your nutritional life.

The Good Mood Diet is the beginning of the rest of your nutritional and emotional life. You will feel great while you lose weight, particularly as you realize your body-fat percentage is lowering. Fact is, you'll probably feel better than you ever have and you'll happily stick to the plan. Once you have lost the weight, you'll have an adaptable nutrition strategy to keep you living at peak levels for a lifetime.

And *nutrition* won't be a negative word in your vocabulary.

Why am I so sure about this? Because this is what I do for my clients every day. Some come to me to lose weight, others want better performance.

I have created diets for athletes for almost twenty-five years. Sports nutrition is all about two things: altering body composition (losing fat and gaining muscle) and staying energized. No matter how great the athlete, it's his or her high mood state that is often the greatest key to success. I have seen it work for pro football linebackers, pro basketball point guards, and Olympians in sports ranging from running to skiing.

Without that food-inspired feeling of exuberance, winning is just a pipe dream. A depressed athlete may as well sit on the sidelines. If they were placed on any of the popular weight-loss diets on the market today, most champions wouldn't get out of the locker room.

Think about that. We wouldn't dream of asking a top athlete to severely restrict calories or tell a child to eat only one meal per day. But that is often common practice for someone trying to lose weight. Why should we fuel our own bodies any less than the quarterback trying to win the Super Bowl or a third-grader who needs to succeed on a spelling test, run hard at recess, and partake in a piano lesson, all during one typical day?

Eating more food, especially at breakfast and mid-morning, can change your life in just a week, maybe sooner.

Here's why: Your body and brain are made of the same atoms, molecules, tissues, and organs as any athlete's. What you need from a diet is the same lift they do — away from depression and toward exuberance. You need to feel great while you lose weight. The Good Mood Diet can get you there.

My Good Mood plan comes from a decade of working with people just like you who were sick of diets that made them feel lousy and didn't work. They were sick of depriving themselves.

"Finally," writes one client in a recent email, "I have a diet plan that doesn't make me feel like I can only choose foods by default, that all the good foods are off-limits. I can't tell you how happy and in control that makes me feel."

I have applied the same principles of sports nutrition and mood-altering food to the diets of my clients who are not athletes. They too want to feel great every day while they lose weight and become more fit. The Good Mood Diet will do that for you, even through the dark days of winter or your own version of deep-freeze periods in your life.

After so many depressing attempts at weight loss, here's your chance to eat food, feel great, and shed the fat you so long have thought would never disappear. That's enough to put anybody in a Good Mood.

Take a drive on the food-and-mood superhighway.

The first step is to understand that all foods affect mood. This chapter highlights the Feel-Great Foods in our lives and pantries. I always like to focus on the positive first. Chapter 2 will review the Feel-Bad Foods. It is a short list — every client is happy to hear that — and some of its items, like chocolate and wine, can even be moved to the Feel-Great list. Then Chapter 3 puts it all together with the Good Mood Menus and laying out the eating plan.

Let's cover a few basics about food and mood. A bit of science will help you understand, for instance, why it is vital to eat the Feel-Great

Foods every day even if you have, well, let's just say strayed from the program a bit.

Ever get a sugar high? Does chocolate make you feel happy and satisfied? Then you've experienced firsthand how food affects mood. We are living during revolutionary times, when scientists are beginning to understand how the brain and the body are linked. Today's advanced imaging technology — PET scans and functional MRIs are two examples — allows researchers to actually watch how the human brain responds to outside stimuli like the food we eat and the activities we pursue.[4]

The brain is the body's control center, but it is integrally linked to the body's responses to external stimuli. What and when we eat directly affects mood. And our mood not only affects what we choose to eat, but how our body responds to that food.

Too often people don't realize that food affects mood every time they eat — in a kitchen, break room, or food court. Let me repeat. Not only *what* but *when* and even *where* we eat directly affect mood. That is one part of the two-way superhighway of nutrition.

In the second lane of this food-mood superhighway, our mood affects what foods we *choose* to eat and how our body *responds* to those foods.

Your brain is profoundly changed with every meal and snack. We will use that physiological fact as a secret ingredient for Good Mood success. You will be feeding both your body and your brain on this plan. You will be treating your moods right and your moods will treat you right back.

Depression is the leading cause of disability in the United States. It can manifest itself in several forms, from major depressive symptoms easily identified as a clinical disorder, to mild chronic symptoms that can persist for several years. According to the National Institute of Mental Health, major depression affects nearly twice as many women (6.7 million) as men. Mild, chronic depressive symptoms affect approximately 5.4 percent of the United States population age eighteen and older at some time during their lifetime. This translates to about 10.9 million American adults. The symptoms often begin in childhood, adolescence, or early adulthood.

Researchers contend that depression is both the most overmedicated (for people with mild depression taking strong medicines) and under-medicated illness in the United States. My take is that following a plan like the Good Mood Diet is a good idea for anyone with mood challenges. It will sort out who really needs pharmaceutical support. Food is mood medicine, plain and straight.

Women who have had an episode of depression have increased odds of developing abdominal obesity, high blood pressure, elevated blood sugar, and unhealthy cholesterol levels. Commonly referred to as *metabolic syndrome,* these conditions set the stage for type 2 diabetes, heart disease, and stroke.

This pattern is not surprising. When you're depressed you don't take care of yourself. Depressed people are more likely to smoke, eat an unhealthy diet, stop exercising, and not comply with medical treatment. They give up on consistency of positive health habits.

Conversely, studies show that obesity increases the risk of depression. So once you are overweight you have a greater chance of becoming depressed, which may thwart any efforts that you make to improve your lifestyle and lose weight: a vicious cycle.

One of my vital Feel-Great Foods might surprise you: fat-free milk.

I think milk has fallen out of favor with too many Americans at the expense of higher rates of depression and mood swings.

If you have sworn off milk for whatever reason — and I find clients who have plenty of reasons for the abstinence — then be open to including it in your diet again. Here is an important distinction: Too many people drink too much milk at one time. That's what causes many of the reactions to milk. Eight ounces or 1 cup is the ideal serving. It might be that 4 to 6 ounces is a better intermediate amount for some individuals. Space out those 8-ounce servings every few hours for optimal energy.

I recommend fat-free organic milk, and everyone who trusts me comes back saying how the milk tasted so good and that drinking only 1 cup or 8 ounces at a time eliminated whatever digestive or sinus problems used to occur.

Whey protein is a naturally rich source of tryptophan. Studies indicate whey can decrease physiological responses to stress, enhance mood, and even improve memory performance. The research on whey is building rapidly; I am very excited about the strong link between whey and enhanced mood.[5]

People who are mildly depressed get the most benefit. Dairy foods are high in whey protein. The best sources are reduced-fat and fat-free milk, yogurt, cottage cheese, and dairy beverages like kefir. Another great source is flavored whey powder, which is the key ingredient in the mid-morning smoothie snack in the Good Mood plan.

Eliminate carbohydrate madness once and for all.

To take license with a popular phrase about the economy: It's the carbohydrates, stupid! Just when everyone is taking aim at carbohydrates and eliminating them from weight-loss diets, these are some of my most critical Feel-Great Foods. For all its positives in your diet, the tryptophan in turkey, dairy, or a good whey protein powder can become a building block of serotonin only after it crosses the blood-brain barrier. Oddly enough — and significantly — it isn't the protein but the dietary carbohydrates in the diet that affects the crossing.

In the bloodstream, the amino acid tryptophan competes with other structurally similar amino acids, called *large neutral amino acids* (LNAA) for a spot on the carrier molecule that transports them across the blood-brain barrier. When protein intake is high, there is an abundance of LNAAs and similar amino acids. Competition for spots is high, limiting tryptophan's access into the brain.

Stay with me here. A breakthrough point comes next. It will allow you to feel guiltless about toast in the morning or a burger bun at night.

When protein intake is lower and carbohydrate intake higher, however, then there is less competition for space on the carrier molecule. In addition, carbohydrates give tryptophan another advantage by stimulating a series of biochemical events that removes most of the LNAA, except for tryptophan, from the bloodstream and placing them into muscle cells. So carbohydrate-rich diets give tryptophan a competitive edge to cross the blood-brain barrier, elevating brain concentrations of serotonin and enhancing mood.

Bottom line: Carbs turn out to be good for you. They do the advance work for proteins. Avoid them because some fad diets claim that they make you fat, and what you do instead is rob Good Mood from your days.

Several studies have documented that diets containing at least 40 percent of calories from carbohydrates can have mood-improving effects on clinically depressed subjects.[6] These diet-induced alterations in mood are less pronounced in healthy subjects since it is more difficult to show the impact of a mood change in someone who isn't markedly depressed. But in my practice, the first thing I hear after clients have followed my program for only one week is, "I have so much more energy, and I feel better than ever!"

I don't mean occasionally. I mean with every new client or the hundreds of *Seattle Post-Intelligencer* readers who followed the Good Mood Diet after it was published. Every time out.

"I want to learn more," wrote one woman. "I lost 5 pounds since last Wednesday [one week's time] but most of all I simply feel like I am a couple of decades younger."

Choose Feel-Great carbs.

When we talk about carbs, we mean whole grains, fruits, vegetables, and legumes. The Feel-Great Foods list on page 15 reviews the Feel-Great Foods in these categories. I recommend getting almost all of your bread servings from the whole-grain group (you can turn pizza into a powerhouse food with a Good Mood whole-wheat crust pizza that even kids will love).

The Good Mood plan is specific about fruits and veggies for optimal energy and happy feelings. I suggest at least one fruit daily from each of the citrus and berry families (use frozen berries in off-season), plus at least one serving each day from the carotene (carrots, dark leafy greens, tomatoes), brassica (broccoli, cauliflower, cabbage, Chinese cabbage, Brussels sprouts), and allium (garlic, onions, shallots, chives) families.

You want to choose foods that your body uses on time-release rather than all at once. Research shows that low- to moderate-glycemic-index carbohydrates are the best choices for control of mood state. High-glycemic-index carbohydrates lead to peaks and valleys in serotonin and mood.

What is the glycemic index? The glycemic index is a scale describing how high your blood sugar rises after digesting a carbohydrate-containing food. Foods on the index are rated numerically, with glucose at 100. In essence, the higher the number assigned to a food, the faster it digests and converts to glucose, and the worse it will make you feel when your blood sugar dips.

Digestion speed is affected by the makeup of a particular food. For instance, a greater amount of fiber, protein, and fat in various foods tends to slow digestion. More of the high-fiber, whole foods are at the low end of the glycemic index, and more refined, processed, and generally sweeter foods are closer to the higher end. Feel-Great Foods in the Good Mood Diet are low to moderate on the glycemic index.

The other half of the glycemic release equation is the portion size. The "load" of carbohydrate that gets into your bloodstream makes a big difference in how your blood sugar, and your mood, responds. So it's not only the choice of food that you make, but also the amount that you eat at one time. That's why the Good Mood Menus so clearly explain not only what food you should eat, but also how much. Within a week to ten days you'll know this stuff like the back of your hand.

A bonus feature of eating low- to moderate-glycemic-index carbohydrates is that they encourage the body to burn and shed fat. You feel less hungry and your body is working to trim the flab. How can you beat that?

Well, as we will discuss in Chapter 6, adding regular exercise will allow you to eat even more food and lose weight easily.

You will always want to combine carbs, protein, and fats in any meal or snack. For instance, a mid-afternoon snack of almonds, dried fruit, and V8 Juice is an ideal pick-me-up and quite satisfying. If you are moderately active (or a male), you can add string cheese to the snack. Enjoy this snack or a variation for one workweek. By Thursday you will feel less blah in the afternoons and by Friday someone will likely comment on your job well done or good points at a meeting.

My friends and family all know they can count on me for healthy snacks. I carry bags around in my car, purse, and even briefcase. Planning your snacks and taking them along with you can change your mood and drop pounds. The Good Mood Traveler chapter (page 118) goes into more detail.

Maximize your success by getting enough fish and flax.

Here's why we need fats in our meals and snacks. Sixty percent of the brain consists of fats. It needs fats to thrive. The Good Mood Diet highlights the right kinds of fats to feed the brain — and your taste buds will be just as tickled.

Polyunsaturated fatty acids (PUFA) in the membranes surrounding brain cells play a role in every step of serotonin function, including boosting mood and keeping it elevated. Serotonin carries messages between brain cells. The term that scientists use to describe a healthy brain cell membrane is *fluid*. We're not talking about water here but lubricating fats. Brain cell membranes must be relatively fluid in order to put the serotonin to work sending messages efficiently and effectively.

It is the concentration of PUFAs in brain cells that determines the fluidity of the membrane. High concentrations of omega-3 fats (a type of PUFA found predominantly in fatty fish) are critical to fluidity.

So eating wild salmon and low-mercury tuna is good for the brain and for your heart. Forget the high fat content. This is healthy fat. Eating these fish will help you lose weight too. New research points to fish oil as the major protector against prostate cancer and other cancers.[7]

The same goes for adding a daily egg and 1 tablespoon of ground flaxseed to your diet. You can use packaged flax meal, but don't settle for eating the whole seeds (about a dollar per pound in bulk). We can't digest the seed hull; the seed's inner goodness and fat-busting qualities will pass right through you. Flaxseed is easy to grind in a coffee-bean grinder. I have a small grinder solely dedicated to flax.

Some people don't like the taste of flax meal, while other clients love the nuttiness mixed right into a bowl of cereal or yogurt with fruit. No matter your taste buds, it is easy to mask in a smoothie, or even blend the flax meal into a scrambled egg or hamburger patty. But I think the best place for it is with your cereal in the morning.

Here's where home recipes meet science. A recent study examining the association between depression and selected nutritional factors found lower levels of omega-3 fats in the red blood cells of depressed women when compared to healthy women. It also found significantly lower levels of alpha-linolenic acid (ALA) and linoleic acid, two essential fatty acids found in flax. These study results support the results of several earlier studies. Fish and flax put you back in balance.[8]

A study conducted in 1998 investigated the influence of total dietary fat on mood. During the first month of the study all subjects ate a diet consisting of 41 percent of the calories from fat. During the second month, half of the subjects switched to a 25-percent-fat diet. Following the second month, levels of anger and hostility increased dramatically in the low-fat group. Tension and anxiety were decreased in the higher fat group.

In addition, a 2006 study followed anger levels in aggressive adults, finding that regular intake of fish oil mellows out even the hard-line personality types.

There's more beyond the mood upswing of the correct fats. HDL cholesterol (the good cholesterol) levels improve on higher-fat diets and decline when a person follows a very low-fat regimen. Remember, salmon, tuna, and other cold-water fish (sardines, anchovies, herring, shellfish) are good for the brain *and* the heart. The Good Mood Diet calls for five servings of fish per week and a daily tablespoon of ground flaxseed.

Plot your WHAT and WHEN strategy.

We will discuss the kinds of meals and snacks in the Good Mood plan, along with when to eat them, in much more detail in Chapter 3 and beyond. But I do want to give you a glimpse here.

The successful strategies of the Good Mood Diet hinge on the critical elements of timing and combining food to get the biggest bang for your buck — for both fat loss and mood control. **The combinations of foods in the Good Mood Menus are as important as the foods themselves.**

Let's be clear and practical about food timing and combining. Every meal and snack needs a balance of carbs, fats, and proteins. Never snack on only carbs, even the fabulous choices of fruits and veggies. Add some nuts or a piece of your favorite cheese. Put protein powder in your smoothies, add flaxseed to your cereal, top toast with almond butter, and smear peanut butter on your crackers.

As for timing, saying you will eat every two to three hours takes planning and forming the habit. You will notice a dramatic rise in energy within the first week of more consistent eating; "no meal-skipping" is your credo. It will take maybe two to three weeks to make it a habit, but it is well worth the adjustment. Some of my clients have lost significant pounds based almost entirely on no longer skipping meals or loading up on the day's calories only at dinnertime and into the evening.

Trust me, this method works. You have to overcome lifelong ideas that eating during the day causes you to gain weight. It is the complete opposite. You will have more energy for life — work, exercise, love interests, shopping, you name it — and rev up your capacity to lose weight. All by simply eating more constantly.

Here's another major lesson I've learned from working with pro and elite athletes across more than a dozen sports: Without enough calories in your diet you will crash and burn early in the day, long before you maximize the amount of food you are eating for peak performance. Athletes who play late-afternoon or evening games need to eat throughout the pre-game part of the day.

This is important: In order to lose weight you need to eat enough calories. Sounds crazy, right? The exercise science experts call it *energy flux.* It basically means your metabolism won't burn at higher rates to shed fat until you increase both food and exercise volume. Exercising more and eating less is a one step forward, two steps back proposition (with apologies to the Bruce Springsteen song).

Bottom line: You need the calories in order to be able to exercise and be physically active. It is the exercise that helps you build muscle. And that newly built muscle burns fat. That's how you lose weight.

Without enough food you wimp out on your exercise plan. You may lose weight on a low-calorie diet, but as we've said, you feel lousy; plus, too much of your weight loss is muscle weight. The moment you fall off the plan, which you will, you'll gain back all you've lost, and likely more in terms of body fat.

How much is enough food? The Good Mood Diet uses a highly scientific strategy to give you just enough of the right kind of calories so that you stay energized all day, feel great, and lose weight. The work of figuring out what and how much is already done for you. The science is built into the plan. Just follow the meal templates, menu plans, and recipes. You'll be feeling better in no time. For the first time, you'll feel great while you lose weight!

A Good Mood Breakthrough Story:

BYE-BYE WEIGHT WATCHERS AND JENNY CRAIG

Many Good Mood Dieters are unsatisfied alumni of high-profile programs, including Weight Watchers, Jenny Craig, and Atkins. They discover an important difference in the Good Mood plan in just days, sometimes even after twenty-four hours.

"I felt good and keep feeling good," exults Louise Goodman, who lost 10 pounds in her first three months in a Good Mood Diet Club. "I could never follow those other diets and plans. I tried pretty much all of them and never stuck with them."

Louise enjoys the Good Mood strategies of eating more nuts and seeds, plus dipping apple slices into peanut butter for an afternoon snack. She also tried turkey jerky for snack time and loves it. She is finding plenty of Good Mood recipes to fit her lifestyle and keeps a bag of frozen cooked chicken breasts and strips to quickly put together a dinner.

"The Good Mood plan is one I will follow for life," Louise says. "It's the first time I have ever connected food to my moods. It works. When I fall off the plan for a day, I notice I feel lousy."

With the other diets, the opposite occurs. On Atkins, for instance, you feel "cranky" while walking the high-protein tightrope and only feel in a good mood when you go off the plan.

"I have absolutely no cravings," says Louise. "That's a miracle in itself for me. I trust the program, and I have never felt this way about a diet before."

2

FEEL-BAD FOODS
(IT'S A SHORT LIST)

Here's one of the best features of the Good Mood Diet: You don't have to eliminate any foods from your eating plan. In fact, I encourage you to include some chocolate and added sugar to your week, along with red wine if you are inclined.

This book is about staying in a Good Mood, remember?

Even so, chances are you will cross off a good number of this chapter's Feel-Bad Foods from your daily menus. That's because you will rapidly understand how foods make you feel. It will become natural to eat more foods from the Feel-Great list in Chapter 1 and choose less frequently from the Feel-Bad list on page 40.

This is a big step that can resonate for a lifetime. You will realize how certain foods in certain portions blitz your mood like a linebacker clobbering a quarterback during a football game. The Good Mood approach is to figure out a way to eat those foods in smaller portions while still enjoying them for the culinary experience and the sheer fun of it.

It's not about eliminating foods you love, but about appreciating them more.

"I came to realize that I was gobbling chocolate chip cookies to stuff down the stress in my life," says Paula Burke, a Seattle-based business consultant with two young children at home. "Now I really savor a good piece of chocolate, taking the time to take pleasure in it. I enjoy it so much more."

A key Good Mood strategy is eating Feel-Great Foods that you enjoy — and that satisfy your hunger.

One example is almonds as part of your mid-afternoon snack. You won't be ravenous at dinner because the nuts satiate your appetite. There are even studies to prove that a pre-dinner snack of nuts will curb your fat consumption at dinner much more dramatically than, say, the seemingly more health-conscious rice cakes.[1]

It works the same way at lunch. You won't be tempted to wolf down a fast-food sandwich and fries — you simply won't feel like doing that — if you follow the Good Mood plan to eat breakfast and then break for a mid-morning smoothie. Plus, you will become aware of your emotional upswing in the hours after a Good Mood lunch. You will want to eat from the Feel-Great list during your workday, at home, on weekends — whenever and wherever you want to feel great.

Let's talk about fried foods to make a vital point. I am not saying that you need to give up eating fish and chips, just that if you do, make sure it is worth the splurge. Perhaps you can split an order with a friend or loved one. And, to repeat my mantra, be sure the day that features a fish-and-chips meal still includes Feel-Great staples such as a whole egg, flax meal, mid-morning smoothie . . . you know the drill.

Similarly, I don't suggest you have to pass on a friend's mother's outrageously good fried chicken. You certainly don't want to offend someone's mama, plus, hey, this is family culture here. Take a piece, savor it, then think about how your body energy is likely to dip, swoon, and crash if you eat three or four pieces of that chicken. Understand your Good Mood margin.

It's uncanny how most of the Feel-Bad Foods are ones that often give immediate gratification, but in the long run make you feel lousy.

The immediate gratification comes from flavors, aromas, and what taste experts call *mouth-feel*. That "long run" might be an hour, the next morning, or over time when you realize you just don't feel that great about your energy level or about yourself. The "comfort" from comfort foods usually doesn't equate to a surge in energy. A nap, maybe, but not more energy.

The popular term "food coma," used liberally during Thanksgiving, refers to a distinct lack of energy resulting from food. The fact is that it is easier to overeat when too large a share of your meals or snacks come from the Feel-Bad list.

Good news, though. The Feel-Bad Foods list is short and even includes some items that qualify for the Feel-Great list in the proper amounts, such as coffee and red wine. Here's the list:

FEEL-BAD FOODS

Alcohol

Caffeine (large doses)

Fried foods

Fatty meats

Fatty snack foods

Refined sugars and starches (most often in packaged foods)

In reasonable amounts, many Feel-Bad Foods can be balanced into meals and even snacks after the first two weeks.

I eliminate Feel-Bad Foods altogether during the Good Mood Accelerator phase (the first two weeks of the Good Mood plan, detailed in Chapter 3) because of the powerful depressive effects of Feel-Bad Foods. I want you to see how great you will feel eating from the Feel-Great list, and then how — as in how much is too much — the Feel-Bad Foods can adversely affect you once you reintroduce them into your diet. Let your mood be your guide, not any diet or menu plan.

The Good Mood Accelerator phase is no gimmick. My clients routinely report feeling more energy within days of starting a program that cuts out the Feel-Bad Foods completely for the first two weeks.

"My energy has been terrific," said Felicity Mansanarez, a thirty-one-year-old nurse at the end of the first week on the Good Mood program. "And it seems, strangely enough, that I have more patience."

Imagine the possibilities. Food affecting your capacity for working better or listening more closely to your loved ones.

Three months into her Good Mood experience, Felicity was even more enthusiastic about both her mood (way up, much more even-keeled) and clothing size (everything was fitting without the usual snugness). She lost 7 pounds and seriously reapportioned her body shape to add more lean muscle and less fat. Felicity wasn't looking to lose lots of pounds, just those elusive last 5 to 8.

Mission accomplished.

Felicity even felt free to share appetizers when out with friends.

"It wasn't fair," she says, smiling. "I would go out with my friends, my skinny friends. They would eat whatever they wanted and not gain weight. I felt like I couldn't eat without gaining pounds. So I was either hungry or guilty about eating."

Felicity endured a significant job change while starting the diet. She adjusted without a problem to starting work at 6:00 a.m. three days a week.

"It's the first time I have woken up without an alarm clock since I was a kid," says Felicity, smiling. "And I am getting up pretty early too."

Let's go through the Feel-Bad list one category at a time. Don't forget, the Good Mood Plan is not about avoiding these foods, but understanding how they make you feel. It is your decision — not any food policing on my part, ugh, I don't even like that word. You alone will determine just how to best navigate the Feel-Bad list for your optimal mood.

Here is an important point: The Good Mood Diet doesn't demand you stop drinking a glass of wine at dinner or sharing a dessert with your family. It is about making conscious choices about what foods lift your mood and help scrub away the depression. Your goal is to feel great, not deprived or suffering from a sugar hangover.

If you want to lose weight, one of the fastest methods is to eliminate alcohol (if you drink it).

There are many who vow to cut back on alcohol a bit, then fail. The reason is not because you drink too much. It's because you expect too much pleasure or escape from that extra glass of wine or the second (or third) cocktail.

Let's just say the research on alcohol and health benefits is, well, fluid. But it is solid that moderate drinking is positive for body weight compared to overdoing it. What's critical is how you define *moderate* when it comes to drinking.

One study by scientists at the Mayo Clinic and Texas Tech University, and published online in the journal *BMC Public Health,* shows that people who have about a drink each day are 54 percent less likely to become obese (measured at 20 percent or more over healthy body weight) than nondrinkers.[2] Among moderate drinkers, half of them were in normal weight range while only a quarter of nondrinkers fit that profile.

Now I am not urging someone to begin consuming alcohol, just reporting that moderate consumption can boost health — and your mood, especially when a glass of red wine and relaxed conversation are your choices.

On the other hand, the same study found consuming four or more drinks daily (48 ounces of beer, 20 ounces of wine, four 1.5-ounce shots) makes a person 46 percent more likely to become obese. Overall, the moderate drinkers who were least likely to become obese or overweight averaged one to two drinks when they consumed, but typically less than five drinks per week.

There is a good case for drinking red wine compared to other forms of alcohol, mostly because it has more antioxidants from the grapes to help prevent heart disease and certain cancers. Dark beer is considered the better choice than lagers for similar reasons. On a practical level, I think that red wine is more a drink you would sip than, say, a cold beer or even cold white wine. It can help people stay in the moderate category.

So, you can see that in moderate amounts wine can switch over to the Feel-Great list. If weight loss is a primary goal, then making the commitment to skip all alcohol for the first two weeks, and then limiting yourself to one to two glasses of wine per week, moves you well on the way to losing pounds. Once you get to your ideal weight, let your mood and energy levels dictate what moderate consumption means for you.

Some of my clients are quite satisfied with a couple glasses of wine each week (and savor them) while others, particularly if they exercise regularly, find that the combination of very regular exercise and the Good Mood Diet lifts their mood so much and makes them feel so good that they don't even want (or need) the sensation that they get from alcohol anymore. They are coping well with the stresses of life, and they don't need to cloud their thoughts to have a good time. They prefer the crystal clear focus and happy mood state of high mental and physical energy, and don't want to feel groggy or foggy from alcohol.

Having given you the research party line on alcohol, let me give you my take, coming from years of practical experience. Yes, alcohol may reduce your stress and relax you, but it also relaxes your inhibitions and increases your appetite. For just about everyone that means that after a drink or two you don't care what or how much you eat anymore: You're living "in the moment." While celebrating like this every once in a while is just fine, if you have long-term goals of raising your mood and losing weight, celebrating on a daily basis will definitely sabotage your plans.

Trish Zuccotti is one of my clients and a top executive at the online travel site Expedia. She and her husband, Andrew, enjoy "really great" wine. They both have noticed how much more energy they feel when following the Good Mood approach to wine. Trish says she feels a particular boost after several days.

"What I have come to realize is I just don't drink run-of-the-mill wine served at a business function or some other gathering," says Trish. "I am more selective."

So I'm asking you to give me two alcohol-free weeks. During that time, enjoy the company that you are in when everyone else is enjoying the alcohol. Replace the ritual of alcohol with something else delicious, like fresh-squeezed juice in a fun cocktail glass or wine glass. We'll talk more about how important rituals are in your life. Rather than just saying "no," we'll give you something just as fun and appealing to enjoy. Before you know it, the wine aficionados will be asking you about what you're drinking and why.

One more note about alcohol. Like the rest of the Good Mood Diet, timing and combining play a role. Always eat before you drink. Eating a shrimp cocktail or other lean protein before having a drink significantly affects absorption of alcohol in the stomach. Food slows transport of the alcohol into the duodenum (your small intestine). The longer alcohol stays in the stomach, the less it can affect you during a party or the next day.

Don't stop drinking coffee or even caffeinated soda, just control your consumption after lunch.

As you read in Chapter 1, caffeinated beverages are actually part of the Feel-Great list. They make the Feel-Bad list only if you consume them in larger amounts.

Here's the Good Mood rule of thumb: If you were a big caffeine user before starting the Good Mood Diet, then continue consuming one to two caffeinated beverages each — but only before noon. After that, switch to green tea if you want a gentle but mood-boosting lift. Drinking more water in the afternoon is another success strategy.

Now, an important question. What qualifies as one to two caffeinated beverages, and what pushes you into the "large doses" category? One to 2 cups of home-brewed coffee (a short or tall cup at Starbucks), one to two shots of espresso, 1 to 2 cups of tea or one to two 12-ounce cans of soda (go diet if you insist on soda) fit the Good Mood parameters.

A large dose is everything above that — though, again, you know best how caffeine affects your mood. Some individuals can handle a bit more caffeine (grande size at Starbucks or 16 ounces), but be honest and alert to what happens when you consume more caffeine than the two-beverage limit. Remember, noon is your caffeine deadline.

Changing your coffee habits takes some planning. Make sure you carry water with you for afternoon breaks and coffee cravings. You might consider carrying a thermos of hot water for green tea if you don't have access to a steaming cup in your day. Experiment with the many varieties of green tea on the market — even going so far as to pick up a few different kinds at an Asian grocery or specialty tea shop. There are even a few great online purveyors that have convenient and delicious loose leaf and bagged teas (try www.teavana.com or www.teaosophy.com). Make it a fun project for yourself and maybe a partner or friend to decide which brand you like best.

Here's the great thing about green tea besides the avalanche of positive research studies about its health benefits[3]: You can drink up to 3 cups in the afternoon (16 to 20 ounces) and boost your mood. If you replace your morning coffee with green tea, then 5 to 7 cups daily is still a Good Mood strategy. You can have your work beverage "fix" and boost your mood too.

Know the power of fried foods and fatty meats.

Everybody knows that deep-fried foods and fatty meats are not going to be a centerpiece of any healthy eating strategy (unless you believe the bacon zealots who follow a high-protein plan that is long on unhealthy portions and the potential for crankiness). But nobody ever talks about the mood power that can be unleashed from fried foods and fatty meats.

It's typically not positive power but still mood-changing. The main reason is because we consume too much fried foods and fatty meats. We overdo it — eating our own super-sized order of fries, consuming four sausages instead of one or two — then feel bad about it emotionally while our physical body comes crashing down too.

In the first two weeks of the Good Mood Accelerator phase, I ask you to eliminate all fried foods and fatty meats to give yourself a baseline of

Good Mood. Then when you move into the second phase of the plan, I ask that you be aware of how these foods make you feel. Don't feel guilty about eating them, please no, but determine how you feel in the hours after eating them.

There is a key distinction to make about fried foods. Know the difference between pan-fried and deep-fried. Pan-fried can fit nicely into the Good Mood Menu plan — if you are preparing a chicken dish or maybe some soy sausages that one of my Good Mood Diet Clubs discovered as breakfast treats — while deep-fried is typically a no-man's land for Good Mood. You might discover that the pan-fried fish or oven-baked French fries are just as fun and satisfying as deep-fried fish and chips. Most of all, your Good Mood will not be fried.

Change your snack style: Eat more.

My clients are always happy to hear that I don't rule out snacks and that in fact the Good Mood Diet relies on them. I want you to enjoy a mid-morning smoothie (or equivalent snack), not miss a mid-afternoon mini-meal, and make sure you drink a hot cocoa before bed.

What I want to change is your snack style. The term *snack* conjures up images of crackers or cookies or chips, maybe a piece of fruit if you are thinking healthier. The Good Mood snack style starts with always making sure you get protein, carbohydrates, and healthy fats with each snack. That rules out most snacks found in vacuum-sealed bags and even disqualifies a lone piece of fruit (all carbs).

The Good Mood Menus in Chapter 3 will take you through fourteen days of snack choices, but here is one regular winning combination that I have used with elite athletes and working mothers alike for years. A small can of vegetable juice (such as V8) is your beverage. Then grab a handful of nuts (maybe 10 to 12 almonds), dried fruit (4 to 5 prunes or apricots or a small box of raisins), and, if you are an active person, one low-fat mozzarella string cheese. Pack these items as you head out for the day and you can bypass the cheese curls or nacho chips from the vending machine.

If you insist that your afternoon apple does the trick of curbing hunger, I am not here to argue against eating fresh fruit. I simply ask that you add some almonds or dip your apple pieces in peanut butter. Then see how you feel in the hour or two after that power snack. You will be surprised, but convinced, that eating more Good Mood foods is better than grabbing a small bag of chips or even fat-free rice cakes (which have no protein or mood-boosting fat benefit).

Fatty snack foods are more about convenience than food preferences. The chips are easy to grab from a machine or quick-mart store, so you buy them. Someone brings cookies to the parents' meeting, so you nibble on one or two — or three.

Members of my Good Mood Diet Clubs are constantly amazed at how much better they feel physically by packing the right snacks versus junk choices. They find they don't miss the "empty calories" and get more energy from nuts, string cheese, or air-popped popcorn.

If you simply don't see life ahead without some junk food or snack chips, my "vice" of choice are soy crisps. Genisoy makes the original chip but several natural grocery chains (including Whole Foods and Trader Joe's) now sell house brands. They come in many flavors and provide all of the fun parts of chip eating — but without the trans fat or lack of protein. Some clients call it the single best surprise of their entire Good Mood plan, that they can eat such delicious crisps, guilt-free. Not only guilt-free, you NEED to eat them. They really do make you feel good.

Bottom line: The Good Mood strategy is about eliminating fatty snack foods, but equally imperative is that you are eating substantial snacks. Don't skip your snacks, including the hot cocoa at night. They are just as essential as breakfast, lunch, and dinner.

I even urge you to think about snacks as mini-meals. For instance, some clients like the option of making an egg-white omelet and a glass of fat-free milk to replace the mid-morning smoothie some days.

The snack-style idea is to make sure you are eating some Good Mood foods at least every three hours, which means finding snacks that you can pack and that satisfy both your hunger and fun factor. You will feel the energy difference.

I don't want you to stop eating, only to start giving more attention to added sugar.

Chances are, you have been told your whole life that the only way to lose weight is to stop eating food — and particularly stop eating your favorite foods.

Let's put that concept on the shelf. To me, one of the best ways to lose weight is to control the amount of added sugar in your meals and snacks. We have prepared an entire appendix (page 217) about the often startling amount of added sugar in packaged and processed foods. While you might guess that cookies are sugar magnets, it is likely you don't know that many brands of fruit yogurt (even all-natural varieties) would blow past the 2 tablespoons of added sugar that you can indulge in twice a week. Eat that yogurt if you must, but it means you have to forgo dessert to stay within the Good Mood parameters. My suggestion is to eat plain yogurt with sliced or diced fruit for the same treat, saving your sugar teaspoons for other sweet treats.

Just about now I suspect some readers are thinking, hey, my cookies in the pantry are low-fat and sugar-free. Or that the pudding in the fridge is nonfat and sugar-free. Even chocolate companies make sugar-free products.

Unless you choose those products on a doctor's recommendation, I say the sugar-free product lines aren't likely to boost mood because they are still loaded with refined carbohydrates.

Let's talk Carbohydrates 101. It's not that all carbs make you fat, it's really the refined carbs (sugars and starches) in packaged and processed foods that crank up your fat-making machinery. Insulin is a vital hormone in muscle-building and energy metabolism. But insulin can also throw extra calories to fat-making in the body. If you eat refined carbs in processed foods, your body's insulin response is overstimulated in an unfortunate way. Instead of sending the refined sugars and carbs into energy metabolism, the rapid spike in insulin level causes the body to go into a preferential fat-storage mode. You get fatter and don't even get the benefits of an energy boost. And forget about a boost in mood.

The alternative is choosing whole foods with unrefined sources of sugars and starches, including fruits, veggies, and whole grains. These types of carbs digest more slowly and insulin doesn't rise so rapidly. Your body responds by sending those types of carbs (which include sugars and starches) to muscles for more energy.

Although sugar only occupies one line of the Feel-Bad list, it is a predominant ingredient in most processed foods. There is no way for you to know how much added sugar is in processed foods because manufacturers withhold that information as closely guarded secrets. So in order for you to take back control over this powerful mood depressor, the Good Mood Diet figures in the number of teaspoons of added sugar that you may include every day so that you can enjoy it, yet also keep feeling your best. That doesn't count the sugar that's naturally found in foods like fruit and milk. *Added* means sugar is an added ingredient.

It's hard to go through life without some added sweetness. Sugar is OK on occasion, but be moderate; your mood will thank you. If you want something extra, opt for a noncaloric sweetener. Splenda is my favorite. It tastes the best and appears to have the least number of reports about adverse side effects.

During supermarket tours with my clients (see page 101 in Chapter 4), we stop to talk about reading the labels of packaged and processed foods. The Good Mood plan allows 24 grams (6 teaspoons) of added sugar twice weekly — that's 48 grams in a week (after you enter the Good Mood Accelerator phase). You can quickly become a Good Mood label reader and make room for dessert in your life. How many times do you hear that from a nutritionist?

Establish rituals and focus less on the Feel-Bad list.

You are looking to relax, draw closer to others, savor life. I propose that you can still enjoy a glass of newly discovered syrah or a handcrafted microbrew at the next backyard barbecue. But that you also use some of the healthy rituals described below to provide the emotional lift we too often expect, at least subliminally, from alcohol.

Personal routines are comforting. They make us feel in control, which in turn reduces stress. The number one reason for stress in our lives is lack of control in situations involving other people.

Rituals are a way to interact with others. Tea ceremonies, and the act of making tea at home, are a classic ritual. It is why Starbucks is so successful: It is a ritual to walk in the door and smell the coffee. We order the same thing just about every time. The faces are familiar and the sounds are reassuring. Most of us have a relationship with our local barista that keeps us coming back.

Social drinking is a ritual. We have a whole culture that has developed around wine. Alcohol is a great icebreaker at parties. The return of the cocktail craze is the reemergence of a ritual with new recipes, beautiful glassware, and dedicated cocktail bars and parties.

The Good Mood Diet is full of healthy, happy rituals: an egg every day, grinding your own flax (or just the ground flaxseed every day), the smoothie snack, the evening cup of cocoa.

I want to add the juice cocktail. Instead of removing the important ritual of sharing a social drink with a friend, we're just going to replace the alcohol with different delicious juice cocktail recipes, serving suggestions, and even party ideas. It can become a family ritual, a diet club ritual, or just an excuse for a good party.

This "mocktail" ritual is something I have developed over time but perfected at a birthday party at the Sambar cocktail bar in Seattle's Ballard neighborhood. Sambar has all sorts of delicious, freshly squeezed juices to mix with other ingredients. Then you can add gin, rum, vodka, you name it.

I order a fresh pineapple juice with mint leaves minus the gin. They serve it in the same cool glass that everyone else has, and I'm just as happy as everyone else is, minus the alcohol. It's fabulous and makes for a great positive approach to eliminating alcohol — something that is good for you and makes you feel good rather than leading you to focus on what you feel you're denying yourself.

A Good Mood Breakthrough Story:

THE SINGLE DAD'S DIET

As a single father with two teenage boys, Benito Cervantes found it hard enough to simply get dinner (and breakfast and lunch and snacks) on the table. His stress level and waistline were getting away from him.

He lost 8 pounds on the Good Mood plan in two months — and, better yet, gained a significant energy boost. That comes in handy with two teens in the household.

"I wake up more refreshed and ready for the day," says Benito, fifty-one, who is a private investigator with a demanding schedule. "My stomach used to get upset when I drank my morning coffee, but that has disappeared."

The benefits resonated for Benito most especially after following the plan for several weeks. "I did not wake up in the middle of the night wanting to drink water or feeling like I needed something to snack on," he recalls. "My clothes fit better almost right away. When I got off the plan for a day or two I really felt it."

A year later, Benito was 12 pounds lighter and involved with a regular and very active workout program. His Good Mood tank is on full pretty much all of the time.

Benito says the Good Mood Diet is family-friendly. "I am introducing meals to my kids that they will actually eat and enjoy," he says. "Our meals used to include lots of [unhealthy] fats and white flour. My meals changed dramatically. My kids' meals are going in that direction with more discussions about the right foods."

Benito says the "best experience" about the diet for him was its simple message: "What I put in my mouth right now will affect me the next hours."

3

THE GOOD MOOD PLAN AND FOURTEEN DAYS OF MENUS

The cover of this book promises three distinct outcomes along the Good Mood timeline:

1. One day to feeling better than yesterday
2. One week to erasing depression
3. One month to losing weight for good

Welcome to the plan and the menus that will achieve those results and a lot more. We will go through the Good Mood Diet plan in detail, step by step, meal by meal, mood boost by mood boost.

One important thing: I talk to my clients about this plan being a black-and-white regimen. For at least two weeks, I recommend "out with the Feel-Bad Foods" and "in with the Feel-Great Foods." This black-and-white approach eliminates the possibility of errors in choices or in amounts. It guarantees the one day/one week/one month outcomes. You will feel better almost immediately and any weight you need to lose will start dropping.

What I ask from you is two absolute, black-and-white weeks. The thrust of the Good Mood Diet is to initiate a two-week learning phase for your body and your lifestyle mindset. I call it the Good Mood Accelerator.

By the end of the first week, you will be feeling much better and most likely will never want to go back to the way you felt before. Trish Zuccotti, a competitive weight lifter and top executive with the Expedia travel web site, couldn't believe how much better she felt after a few days even after an adulthood of working out and trying to eat right.

"I just couldn't get over how much more energy I had for workouts — and at the office," recalls Trish.

My Good Mood Diet Club meetings echo the theme. Jennifer Lail from the original newspaper group said her first night's sleep after starting the plan was her best in years, happily followed by many others. Sharon Lee Hamilton, another group member, said she was less stressed around her young children.

After a week, Jennifer said she sensed a distinct lifting of a long-time mild depression. Other clients have confided the same feeling, sometimes flat-out gushing about the change fueled by the black-and-white Good Mood Accelerator.

The funny thing? Many clients and, yes, readers of this book, start the program because of a strong motivation to lose weight. The Good Mood Accelerator rapidly puts you in that body change mode. You will lose fat and gain muscle. You will drop pounds. But the main reason you will stick with the plan won't be linked to the bathroom scale. The main reason will be because you feel good. If you feel good, you stick to the plan. If you stick to the plan, you lose weight. It's that easy.

After the first two weeks in the Good Mood Accelerator phase, you can either stay on that regimen or add back some Feel-Bad Foods that can actually boost mood in the right amounts. I call this option the Feel Great While You Lose Weight phase.

The Good Mood Accelerator is nutritionally sound on a long-term basis. You've only eliminated Feel-Bad Foods. I have some clients who use the Good Mood Accelerator until they lose all of their target weight or reach performance goals or both. Another effective strategy is to reintroduce the Good Mood Accelerator phase into your diet every three to six months, or whenever you feel a need for a mood boost. Some of my clients use it during intense times of work projects to generate energy and better performance.

Many more clients opt for the more relaxed Feel Great While You Lose Weight phase. They are happy to selectively add back some foods and especially eager to try out my position that some chocolate, red wine, or even 6 teaspoons of added sugar twice a week can keep you on plan while improving mood.

Let's get started with the plan by discussing overall guidelines or what I call the Good Mood Template. Then we will go through fourteen days (two weeks) of menus to give you solid ideas about how to prepare meals, dine out, and eat on the go.

The Good Mood Template

Memorize the Good Mood Template or carry the list with you.

Many of my clients make a copy (handwritten or photocopied) of the Good Mood Template. The template outlines the breakdown of food groups, amounts, and combinations for each day's meals and snacks. You will come to memorize the template by following it, particularly during the first two weeks of the Good Mood Accelerator.

First, pick your group for the Good Mood Template.

For purposes of this book, I have divided people into three groups corresponding with the number of calories consumed and level of activity. It is most valuable for you to decide which group fits your goals. Remember that you can shift to another group or calorie level as your lifestyle changes.

Group 1 is for women who want to lose weight or flab and who engage in a moderately active lifestyle (translation: you don't exercise as much as you would like). Group 1 calls for 1,600 calories per day.

Group 2 covers men who want to lose weight or flab and who engage in a moderately active lifestyle. It also includes women who started on the

Group 1 plan but realize they are still hungry, say, mid-morning or mid-afternoon, especially if they are regularly working out at a pretty intense level. The Group 2 regimen calls for 1,800 calories per day. Some men who start in this group may decide to move to Group 3 once they lose weight and/or step up their exercise routines, while others like the built-in weight control effect of Group 2.

Group 3 is a 2,200-calorie-per-day plan that is best suited for highly active people. I have used it for years with elite athletes, including professional football and basketball players, plus Olympians in many sports, although their calorie levels are even higher. It is important for people in Group 3 to time snacks and meals to optimize workout energy and recovery from exercise. Chapter 6 will discuss this important rest and recovery factor.

How the Good Mood Template fits into your life.

The template is basically a set of numbers that is shorthand in your eating plan. You can keep it to one sheet. Some clients convert it into a tally list to be clear in the early days and weeks that they are getting the right foods. It all becomes second nature in a short time. You will soon easily recognize what comprises a Good Mood breakfast, lunch, dinner, or snack.

Here is the template and its basic rules, including specific guidelines for the Good Mood Accelerator and Feel Great While You Lose Weight phases, followed by a summary list of what qualifies for each food group. You can find an expanded list of foods in each food group — bread serving, fat, very lean protein, etc. — in Appendix A on page 205. The chapter finishes with fourteen days of detailed menus and my Real Life notes.

The Good Mood Template: Meals and Snacks

If you follow this pattern of meals and snacks each day, you will optimize mood and weight loss. To accommodate life, you can certainly swap meals when necessary, or move a dinner fruit to flavor your smoothie. But this template is based on years of success with clients and numerous scientific studies on muscle and brain performance. Eating these combinations at the specified times — not going more than two-and-a-half to three hours without food — will make a palpable difference in your energy and outlook.

Breakfast

Group 1	Group 2	Group 3
1 bread	1 bread	2 breads
1 fruit	1 fruit	1 fruit
1 milk	1 milk	1 milk
1 medium-fat protein	1 medium-fat protein	1 medium-fat protein
1 fat	1 fat	1 fat
water	water	water

Morning Snack

Group 1	Group 2	Group 3
1 milk	1 milk	1 milk
2 very lean proteins	2 very lean proteins	3 very lean proteins
		1 fruit

Lunch

Group 1	Group 2	Group 3
1 bread	2 breads	2 breads
2 vegetables	2 vegetables	2 vegetables
3 very lean proteins	4 very lean proteins	4 very lean proteins
1 fat	1 fat	2 fats
water	water	water

Afternoon Snack

Group 1	Group 2	Group 3
1 fruit	1 fruit	1 fruit
1 vegetable	2 vegetables	2 vegetables
1 fat	2 fats	2 fats
	1 very lean protein	2 very lean proteins

Dinner

Group 1	Group 2	Group 3
2 breads	2 breads	2 breads
1 fruit	1 fruit	1 fruit
2 vegetables	2 vegetables	2 vegetables
4 lean proteins	4 lean proteins	5 lean proteins
2 fats	2 fats	2 fats
water	water	water

Evening Snack

Group 1	Group 2	Group 3
1 milk	1 milk	1 milk

Basic Rules of the Good Mood Template

1. Have one whole egg or one daily serving of whole soy such as edamame, tofu, or soy milk every day (use more soy and less egg if you have high cholesterol or a family history of heart disease).
2. Have a serving of nuts (or nut oil) every day.
3. Eat fish five times each week. Make that your goal.
4. Eat a variety of vegetables, including items from the carotene-rich, brassica, and allium families each day (see page 205 in Appendix A). This is different from most eat-your-veggies advice — and will jump-start your mood and weight loss. Note: starchy vegetables such as corn and potatoes count as Good Mood bread servings.
5. Eat a variety of fruits, including servings from the citrus and berries groups each day. These two fruit groups are superpowers.
6. Drink 5 to 6 cups of water every day and 9 to 11 cups fluids in total. This includes moderate amounts of coffee, plus green tea.[1] Keep to no more than one fruit juice serving (4 ounces) most days; switch to vegetable juice for afternoon pick-me-ups.
7. Take one multivitamin-mineral supplement daily, with 100 percent of the minimum for major nutrients based on your age and gender.

Food Groups: Explaining the Good Mood Template Shorthand

Here is a short review of what I mean by each food group and the relative serving sizes. There is an expanded list of these foods by category in Appendix A.

Food Group	Serving Size
Bread	1 slice bread; ½ cup cooked cereal, pasta, or starchy vegetable (such as potatoes or peas); ½ cup rice; 1 ounce ready-to-eat cereal; ½ bun, bagel, or English muffin; 1 small roll; 3 to 4 small or 2 large crackers
Fruit	1 small to medium fresh fruit; ½ cup canned or fresh fruit or fruit juice; ½ cup dried fruit; ½ grapefruit; 1 melon wedge
Milk	1 cup fat-free or 1-percent reduced-fat milk, soy milk, or plain yogurt
Vegetable	½ cup cooked vegetables or vegetable juice; 1 cup raw vegetables
Very lean protein	1 ounce white meat skinless poultry; 1 ounce cod, flounder, haddock, halibut, trout, fresh tuna, or canned tuna in water; 1 ounce shellfish; 1 ounce cheese with less than 1 gram fat per ounce; 1 ounce processed sandwich meats with less than 1 gram fat per ounce; 2 egg whites
Lean protein	1 ounce USDA Select or Choice grades of lean beef, pork, lamb, or veal, trimmed of fat; 1 ounce skinless dark-meat poultry or white-meat chicken with skin; 1 ounce oysters, salmon, catfish, sardines, canned tuna in oil; ¼ cup (4.5 percent) cottage cheese, 2 tablespoons grated Parmesan, 1 ounce cheese with less than 3 grams fat per ounce; 1 ounce processed sandwich meat with less than 3 grams fat per ounce

Medium-fat protein	1 ounce most kinds of beef, pork, lamb, veal, trimmed of fat; 1 ounce dark-meat chicken with skin, ground turkey, or ground chicken; 1 ounce any fish product; 1 ounce cheese with less than 5 grams fat per ounce; 1 whole egg; ¼ cup tempeh, ½ cup (4 ounces) tofu
Fat	1 teaspoon butter, margarine, vegetable oil; 1 tablespoon regular salad dressing; 2 tablespoons reduced-fat salad dressing; 1 tablespoon reduced-fat mayonnaise; 1 teaspoon regular mayonnaise; 2 tablespoons reduced-fat cream cheese; ⅛ medium avocado; 8 olives; 6 to 10 nuts; 2 teaspoons peanut butter or tahini; 1 tablespoon seeds

Serving Totals for the Good Mood Template

Here's what a day of the food group servings looks like:

	Number of Servings		
	Group 1	**Group 2**	**Group 3**
Bread	4	5	6
Fruit	3	3	4
Milk	3	3	4
Vegetable	5	6	6
Very lean protein	5	7	9
Lean protein	4	4	5
Medium-fat protein	1	1	1
Fat	5	6	8

Good Mood Accelerator: The First Two Weeks

To enhance weight loss and mood, include green tea and cocoa powder every day. You can drink up to 3 cups of green tea if you keep drinking coffee or 5 daily cups if you eliminate coffee. Both help the body to burn fat more effectively and just feel better.

Here are items to eliminate completely for just two weeks (remember, keep it black and white for optimal mood and weight loss): Eliminate alcohol, caffeine in large doses, fried foods, fatty meats, refined sugars and starches (mostly found in processed foods, even "healthy" ones). Do not add any table sugar for these first two weeks.

An important note about coffee and caffeine: If you are a big caffeine user, consume one to two caffeinated beverages before noon each day. For example, here are some possibilities:

1 to 2 cups home-brewed coffee or 1 tall Starbucks coffee

1 to 2 shots espresso coffee

1 to 2 cups black tea

1 to 2 caffeinated soft drinks (12 ounces each)

Feel Great While You Lose Weight Phase: Week Three and Beyond

If you would like, after two weeks you can add two servings total of wine, chocolate, and/or added sugar back to your diet — in moderation. If you perceive any negative impact to mood, eliminate the foods again. Keep it to a maximum of two servings total per week for best weight-loss results. Here are what the servings look like:

5 ounces wine (red preferred)

⅔ ounce chocolate (dark preferred)

6 teaspoons added sugar

Here are some week-by-week examples of how to add back and mix and match two servings of treats each week, after the first two weeks of the Good Mood Accelerator:

Week One of the Feel Great While You Lose Weight phase
Sunday afternoon: ⅔ ounce chocolate
Friday night: 5 ounces red wine

Week Two of the Feel Great While You Lose Weight phase
Wednesday night: ⅔ cup fat-free frozen yogurt (6 teaspoons added sugar)
Saturday night: ⅔ ounce chocolate candy

Week Three of the Feel Great While You Lose Weight phase
Thursday afternoon: 1 cup sherbet or sorbet (12 teaspoons added sugar)

Good Mood for a Lifetime

Once you reach your weight goals, let your mood be the best guide for adding back any foods from the Feel-Bad list. I don't have many clients who completely abandon the template because they feel too good following it. They realize how much is too much in terms of chocolate or alcohol.

OK, so let's say that a certain wedding or romantic dinner has surpassed your chocolate and red wine allotment for the week. I hope you enjoyed the splurge. Don't sweat it too much. Just get back on track the next day. Step back on the Good Mood Accelerator for the next few days and notice how it improves your mood and life enjoyment compared to the morning after the wedding or dinner. Let your mood be your guide.

Fourteen Days of Good Mood Diet Menus

Become familiar with these sample menus.

The Good Mood Diet is all about what works with your life. The following pages outline fourteen days of sample menus, complete with three

Free Foods and Drinks That Make You Feel Good

These are foods and drinks that can fit into any day without counting as any calories:

Cocoa powder, unsweetened (1 tablespoon)

Coffee (up to 2 cups per day)

Diet soft drink (up to 2 servings per day, if you insist)

Green tea (up to 5 cups per day; keep it to 3 if you drink coffee)

Flat, sparkling, or mineral water (flavored or plain without sugar)

Nonstick cooking spray

Salsa (½ cup)

Seasonings and herbs

Sugar substitutes (use in moderation)

Turkey broth or consommé

Whipped topping (1 tablespoon)

Wine (used in cooking)

Yogurt (2 tablespoons)

meals, two snacks, and an evening cocoa each day. Feel free to customize your own Good Mood plan. There are three dozen recipes in Chapter 8 to help with your menu planning — and to show that good food can be prepared within minutes in many cases.

Fourteen days of menus allows you to develop a strong habit of Good Mood meals and snacks. I have included Real Life comments for each meal and snack to provide some insights into how these Good Mood meals fit into busy schedules and family eating.

These menus will help you get into a daily rhythm of eating and connecting mood to food. It never fails that at each meeting of my Good Mood Diet Clubs members come up with their own variations or "riffs" on how to plan out daily menus.

One example of variations relates to the first meal of the day. I tend to eat the same breakfast most days, while other Good Mood participants appreciate the choices. There are some people who switch breakfast with the mid-morning smoothie to make a smoother transition from a lifetime of never eating before noontime.

Tailor your menu according to your goals.

These menus are detailed for Group 1, or women who are looking to lose weight or flab while leading a moderately active lifestyle. Group 2 (men looking to lose flab or weight, and women with weight-loss goals and highly active lifestyles) and Group 3 (highly active people not looking to lose weight) both need to add calories to control hunger while fueling the body and a better mood. My clients typically add these extra servings right into their templates and sample menus. If you are not in Group 1, you should add the following to the menus:

Group 2 (1,800-calorie diet) Additions to Each Daily Menu
Lunch: 1 bread, 1 very lean protein
Afternoon snack: 1 vegetable, 1 fat, 1 very lean protein

Group 3 (2,200-calorie diet) Additions to Each Daily Menu
Breakfast: 1 bread
Morning snack: 1 very lean protein, 1 fruit
Lunch: 1 bread, 1 very lean protein, 1 fat
Afternoon snack: 1 vegetable, 1 fat, 2 very lean proteins
Dinner: 1 lean protein

The Good Mood Diet Menus

The following menus are for people in Group 1 or at 1,600 calories per day. If you are in Group 2 or 3, refer to the lists of added servings above. Remember that women who are moderately active and want to lose weight are in Group 1. Men who are moderately active and want to lose weight fit into Group 2. If you become more highly active and hit your weight goals, then be sure to move yourself up at least one group for weight maintenance and optimal energy.

Day 1

Breakfast

1 bread	½ cup shredded wheat or 1 cup Kashi low-sugar cereal
1 fruit	2 tablespoons raisins (or ½ cup blueberries in season)
1 milk	1 cup fat-free milk
1 medium-fat protein	1 egg (cooked any way without fat)
1 fat	1 tablespoon ground flaxseed
	water

Morning Snack

1 milk, 2 very lean proteins	Homemade smoothie: Blend until smooth 1 cup fat-free milk, 14 grams protein from flavored isolated whey protein powder, and 3 ice cubes (Group 3 or highly active people at a healthy weight use 21 grams protein from whey protein powder)

*Measure out the whey powder by determining the size of the scoop supplied with the product, then determine what fraction of scoop equals 14 grams.

Lunch

1 bread	1 cup chicken/vegetable noodle soup
2 vegetables, 1 fat	2 cups mixed green salad with 2 tablespoons reduced-fat olive oil and balsamic vinegar dressing
3 very lean proteins	3 ounces turkey
	water

Afternoon Snack

1 fruit	1 apple
1 vegetable	½ cup vegetable or tomato juice
1 fat	10 peanuts (ballpark-style take longer to eat!)
	water

Dinner

1 bread	½ cup brown rice
1 bread	½ cup baked sweet potato
1 fruit	1 orange
2 vegetables	1 cup steamed broccoli, sprinkled with balsamic or raspberry vinegar
4 lean proteins, 1 fat	4 ounces grilled or broiled wild salmon, rubbed with 1 teaspoon extra-virgin olive oil
1 fat	8 large black olives
	water

Evening Snack

1 milk	Hot cocoa: 1 cup heated fat-free milk mixed with 1 to 2 rounded teaspoons cocoa powder and Splenda to taste.

Real Life: Coffee

I didn't list coffee, but trust me, it is OK to include one to two cups or one to two shots of espresso any time during the morning. I actually eat my egg and drink my coffee when my children wake up, which is about an hour after I eat my usual shredded wheat, flax, and raisins.

Day 2

Breakfast

1 bread, 1 medium-fat protein	½ toasted whole-wheat English muffin, with 1 poached egg
1 milk, 1 fruit, 1 fat	1 cup fat-free unsweetened yogurt with 1 small banana, sliced (or 1 cup berries in season) and 1 tablespoon ground flaxseed
	water

Morning Snack

1 milk, 2 very lean proteins, 1 fruit (fruit serving taken from dinner)	Homemade orange smoothie: Blend until smooth 1 cup fat-free milk, 14 grams protein from flavored isolated whey protein powder, ½ cup orange juice, and 3 ice cubes

Lunch

1 bread	½ cup brown rice
2 vegetables, 3 very lean proteins, 1 fat	Chicken stir-fry: 1 cup Chinese vegetables, garlic, onion, ginger, and 3 ounces white-meat chicken, stir-fried in 1 teaspoon peanut oil
	green tea

Afternoon Snack

1 fruit	1 pear
1 vegetable, 1 fat	1 cup mini-carrots with 2 tablespoons reduced-fat ranch dressing
	water

Dinner

2 breads, 1 vegetable	1 cup cooked whole-wheat pasta topped with ½ cup ratatouille
1 vegetable, 2 fats	Tossed salad with 1 cup lettuce, ½ cup chopped tomato, ½ cup sliced cucumber, ⅛ avocado (sliced), and 2 tablespoons reduced-fat salad dressing
4 lean proteins	4 ounces grilled or broiled lean meat (beef, pork, lamb, dark-meat poultry)
(fruit serving used at morning snack)	water

Evening Snack

1 milk	Hot cocoa: 1 cup heated fat-free milk mixed with 1 to 2 rounded teaspoons cocoa powder and Splenda to taste

Real Life: Takeout

It's hard to find a takeout stir-fry that matches your lunch serving. The first strategy is to find a restaurant that doesn't overdo it on the oil. If you're lucky, you may be able to find one that also offers brown rice — a good barometer of health-conscious cooking.

When you do get stir-fry takeout, figure on saving half or more of the container for the next day's lunch. If you share a refrigerator at work, invest a few dollars in an air-tight container that you like with your name clearly marked. Look for one that is microwave-safe for easy heating.

Day 3

Breakfast

1 bread, 1 medium-fat protein, 1 fat	½ cup cooked oats (not instant) mixed with ½ cup diced tofu, 1 tablespoon ground flaxseed, and Splenda to taste
1 fruit	1¼ cups whole strawberries, sliced (or 1 diced apple if berries are not in season)
1 milk	1 cup fat-free milk
	water

Morning Snack

1 milk	1 cup fat-free milk
2 very lean proteins	Omelet made with 4 egg whites

Lunch

1 bread	1 slice whole-grain bread
2 vegetables, 3 very lean proteins, 1 fat	Tuna salad: 2 cups mixed greens with tomato, red pepper, hearts of palm (if desired), 3 ounces tuna fish (packed in water), and 2 tablespoons reduced-fat olive oil and balsamic vinegar dressing
	water

Afternoon Snack

1 fruit	½ cup dried cherries
1 vegetable	½ cup vegetable or tomato juice
1 fat	10 dry-roasted almonds
	water

Dinner

1 bread, 1 fat	2-inch cube corn bread
1 bread, 1 fat	½ cup mashed potatoes with 1 teaspoon butter or olive oil
1 fruit	½ grapefruit, sprinkled with cinnamon and Splenda to taste and lightly broiled
2 vegetables	1 cup steamed asparagus or green beans, sprinkled with balsamic or raspberry vinegar
4 lean proteins	4 ounces dark-meat turkey
	water

Evening Snack

1 milk	Hot cocoa: 1 cup heated fat-free milk mixed with 1 to 2 rounded teaspoons cocoa powder and Splenda to taste

Real Life: Broiled Grapefruit

Don't knock the broiled grapefruit until you've tried it!

Real Life: Canned Tuna

My favorite canned tuna comes from the company Fishing Vessel St. Jude. It's mercury-free, high in omega-3 fats, and tastes like fresh fish. It is more than worth the extra few dollars. You can find St. Jude on the Web, www.tunatuna.com. There are other entrepreneurial companies now seizing the opportunity to market low-mercury tuna. If you can't get a hold of these, remember that the federal government says light tuna is actually a safer health bet than solid white or albacore.

Day 4

Breakfast

1 bread, 1 fat	½ cup shredded wheat or 1 cup Kashi cereal with 1 tablespoon ground flaxseed
1 fruit	2 tablespoons raisins (or ¾ cup blueberries in season)
1 milk	1 cup fat-free milk
1 medium-fat protein	1 egg (cooked any way without fat)
	water

Morning Snack

1 milk, 2 very lean proteins	Homemade smoothie: Blend until smooth 1 cup fat-free milk, 14 grams of protein from flavored isolated whey protein powder, and 3 ice cubes

Lunch

1 bread, 3 very lean proteins, ½ fat, 1 vegetable	Open-faced lox sandwich: 1 slice whole-grain bread, 3 ounces lox or smoked salmon, 1 tablespoon reduced-fat cream cheese, and sliced cucumber, tomato, and onion
½ fat	4 large black olives
1 vegetable	1 cup carrot sticks
	water

Afternoon Snack

1 fruit	1 apple
1 vegetable	½ cup vegetable or tomato juice
1 fat	10 peanuts (ballpark-style take longer to eat!)
	water

Dinner

2 breads, 2 fats	1 cup whole wheat pasta, tossed with 1¼ tablespoons pesto
4 lean proteins	4 ounces grilled chicken strips
2 vegetables	2 cups sliced cucumber, carrots, celery, and cherry tomatoes
1 fruit	1¼ cups fresh strawberries with 1 tablespoon full-fat whipped topping (free)
	water

Evening Snack

1 milk	Hot cocoa: 1 cup heated fat-free milk mixed with 1 to 2 rounded teaspoons cocoa powder and Splenda to taste

Real Life: Whole-Wheat Pasta

It took a while, but now even my kids eat whole-wheat pasta.

Real Life: Whey Protein

Whey protein in a smoothie is perfect for after exercise. Called a "fast protein," it is digested and absorbed very rapidly, helping your muscles repair, recover, and grow for another hard workout tomorrow. Drink the smoothie as soon after a morning workout as possible: Within thirty minutes is best. It will fuel you up for the rest of your day — no more hitting the wall at 4:00 p.m.

The flavored whey powders offer enough sweetener for most tastes. You can also add one of your fruit servings from other parts of the day to the mid-morning smoothie for sweetness and flavor.

Day 5

Breakfast

1 bread	1 slice whole-grain bread, toasted
1 fruit, 1 milk, 1 medium-fat protein, 1 fat	Mango smoothie: Combine until smooth ½ peeled and chopped fresh mango (or ½ cup frozen mango), 1 cup fat-free milk, 4 ounces silken tofu, 1 tablespoon flaxseed meal, and Splenda to taste
	water

Morning Snack

1 milk	1 cup fat-free milk
2 very lean proteins	omelet made with 4 egg whites

Lunch

1 bread, 1 very lean protein	1 cup bean soup
2 vegetables, 2 very lean proteins, 1 fat	Tuna salad: 2 cups mixed greens, 2 ounces tuna fish, and 2 tablespoons reduced-fat olive oil and balsamic vinegar dressing
	water

Afternoon Snack

1 fruit	1 orange
1 vegetable, 1 fat	1 cup mini-carrots with 1 tablespoon natural peanut butter
	water

Dinner

1 bread	½ cup wild rice
1 bread	½ cup cooked acorn squash
1 vegetable, 1 fat	½ cup asparagus, drizzled with balsamic or raspberry vinegar and 1 teaspoon extra-virgin olive oil
4 lean proteins, 1 vegetable	4 ounces dark meat turkey with ⅓ cup Holiday Cranberry Sauce (page 178)
1 fat	8 large black olives
1 fruit	2 medium fresh figs
	water

Evening Snack

1 milk	Hot cocoa: 1 cup heated fat-free milk mixed with 1 to 2 rounded teaspoons cocoa powder and Splenda to taste

Real Life: Fresh Figs

The first time I had a fresh fig we picked it off a tree in Greece. The delectable tastes are uplifting for your mind and your body. Keep this in mind: We crave dessert not because we are hungry but because we yearn for different taste sensations, such as sweetness. You can choose to save the figs as the final part of your meal to satisfy your sweet tooth.

Real Life: Peanut Butter

Yes, you have permission to add peanut butter back into your diet. It is a comfort food full of wonderful healthy fats and protein. Choose a natural brand; my favorite is Adams. There's no sugar or other additives: just peanuts and salt. It's even available at warehouse stores.

Day 6

Breakfast

1 bread, 1 fat	1 corn tortilla, toasted, with 1 teaspoon Smart Balance Omega-3 spread and garlic salt
1 fruit	⅓ of a cantaloupe
1 milk	1 cup fat-free milk
1 medium-fat protein	1 scrambled egg with 2 tablespoons salsa (free)
	water

Morning Snack

1 milk, 2 very lean proteins	Homemade smoothie: Blend until smooth 1 cup fat-free milk; 14 grams of protein from flavored isolated whey protein powder, and 3 ice cubes
1 fruit (fruit serving taken from dinner)	½ cup frozen mango

Lunch

1 bread, 2 vegetables, 3 very lean proteins, 1 fat	Subway Turkey Breast Wrap: 1 wrap, selection of vegetables, 3 ounces turkey, 1 teaspoon mayonnaise, and Dijon mustard (free)
	water

Afternoon Snack

1 fruit	1 apple
1 vegetable	½ cup vegetable or tomato juice
1 fat	10 peanuts (ballpark-style take longer to eat!)
	water

Dinner

2 breads	1 cup potato-leek soup
2 vegetables	1 cup steamed broccoli, sprinkled with fat-free Italian dressing
4 lean proteins, 2 fats	4 ounces tilapia, brushed with 1 teaspoon olive oil, sprinkled with 1 tablespoon ground flaxseed and ½ teaspoon sesame seeds, and grilled; serve with 2 tablespoons salsa (free)
(fruit serving used at morning snack)	water

Evening Snack

1 milk	Hot cocoa: 1 cup heated fat-free milk mixed with 1 to 2 rounded teaspoons cocoa powder and Splenda to taste

Real Life: Subway

My favorite fast food stop is Subway. The wraps fit the 1 bread and 3 protein servings perfectly for lunch, and you can fill them up with veggies. Choose from any of the wraps listed under the "6 grams of fat or less" category. If you go with a 6-inch sandwich, count it as 3 bread servings and 2 very lean protein servings. Skip the cheese unless you have an extra fat serving to spend. To boost protein, ask for a double serving of the protein filling.

Day 7

Breakfast

1 bread, 1 medium-fat protein	½ toasted whole-wheat English muffin with 1 poached egg
1 milk, 1 fruit, 1 fat	1 cup fat-free unsweetened yogurt, with 1 small banana, sliced (or 1 cup berries in season) and 1 tablespoon ground flaxseed
	water

Morning Snack

1 milk, 2 very lean proteins	Homemade smoothie: Blend until smooth 1 cup fat-free milk, 14 grams of protein from flavored isolated whey protein powder, and 3 ice cubes

Lunch

1 bread, 2 vegetables, 3 very lean proteins, 1 fat	Chicken taco: 1 crispy taco shell, stuffed with shredded lettuce, chopped tomatoes, peppers, 3 ounces chicken, 2 tablespoons sour cream, and 2 tablespoons salsa (free)
	water

Afternoon Snack

1 fruit	1 apple
1 vegetable	½ cup vegetable or tomato juice
1 fat	6 dry-roasted almonds
	water

Dinner

2 breads, 4 lean proteins, 1 vegetable	1 hamburger: 1 small whole-wheat hamburger bun, with 4 ounces grilled chopped sirloin, lettuce, tomato, onion, pickle, and mustard and 1 tablespoon ketchup (free)
1 vegetable, 1 fat	1 cup tossed salad with 2 tablespoons reduced-fat salad dressing
1 fat	8 black olives
1 fruit	17 grapes
	water

Evening Snack

1 milk	Hot cocoa: 1 cup heated fat-free milk mixed with 1 to 2 rounded teaspoons cocoa powder and Splenda to taste

Real Life: Nightly Cocoa

I really look forward to my cup of cocoa at the end of the day, whether it's winter or summer. It's my personal moment of relaxation and reflection; a time to focus on how I feel, how my day went, and what my plan is for tomorrow. I have found that there is no substitute for a good plan — or good chocolate.

I have yet to meet a client that doesn't fall in love with this calming bedtime snack. Even the guys love it.

Day 8

Breakfast

1 bread, ½ milk, 1 medium-fat protein, 1 fat	French toast: Soak 1 slice whole-wheat bread in ½ cup fat-free milk, 1 egg, 1 tablespoon ground flaxseed, and ½ teaspoon cinnamon; cook in a nonstick pan with cooking spray, pouring the remaining egg mixture over the bread.
½ milk, 1 fruit	½ cup fat-free unsweetened yogurt with 1 cup raspberries
	water

Morning Snack

1 milk, 2 very lean proteins, 1 fruit (fruit serving taken from dinner)	Homemade strawberry smoothie: Blend until smooth 1 cup fat-free milk, 14 grams protein from flavored isolated whey protein, 3 ice cubes, and 1¼ cups frozen strawberries

Lunch

1 bread, 1 very lean protein	½ cup kidney beans
2 vegetables, 1 fat	2 cups mixed green salad with 2 tablespoons reduced-fat olive oil and balsamic vinegar dressing
2 very lean proteins	2 ounces turkey
	water

Afternoon Snack

1 fruit	1 apple
1 vegetable	½ cup vegetable or tomato juice
1 fat	1 tablespoon tamari-roasted sunflower seeds
	water

Dinner

2 breads, 1 fat, 4 lean proteins, 2 vegetables	Smoked-fish sandwich: 1 whole-wheat bagel with 2 tablespoons reduced-fat mayonnaise, 4 ounces Smoked-Fish Pâté (page 158), lettuce leaf, sliced tomato, cucumber, onion, and pickle
1 fat	8 black olives
(fruit serving used at morning snack)	water

Evening Snack

1 milk	Hot cocoa: 1 cup heated fat-free milk mixed with 1 to 2 rounded teaspoons cocoa powder and Splenda to taste

Real Life: Turkey

Turkey is a very lean protein food that is high in tryptophan. It will pick you up and reduce your anxiety, especially on those very stressful days.

Real Life: Vegetable Juice

A mini-can of vegetable or tomato juice makes for a great portable snack. You can easily pack it in your purse or briefcase.

Real Life: Berries

When it comes to fruits, berries are one of the best deals in town. Not only are they incredibly delicious and nutritious, but you get a huge serving for one portion. Use frozen in off-season; watch for sales and stock up.

Day 9

Breakfast

1 bread, 1 fat	½ cup cooked oatmeal with 1 tablespoon ground flaxseed
1 fruit	½ cup orange juice
1 milk	1 cup fat-free milk
1 medium-fat protein	2 Morningstar Farm Veggie Breakfast Sausage Links
	water

Morning Snack

1 milk, 2 very lean proteins	Homemade smoothie: Blend until smooth cup fat-free milk, 14 grams of protein from flavored isolated whey protein powder, and 3 ice cubes

Lunch

1 bread, 3 very lean proteins, 1 fat	1 slice (⅛ of 12-inch pie) thin-crust BBQ chicken and cheese pizza
2 vegetables	2 cups mixed green salad with 2 tablespoons fat-free salad dressing
	water

Afternoon Snack

1 fruit	½ cup grapefruit juice
1 vegetable, 1 fat	1 cup mini-carrots with 2 tablespoons reduced-fat ranch dressing
	water

Dinner

2 breads	2 slices crusty French bread
2 vegetables, 1 fruit, 2 fats	Spinach salad: 2 cups spinach with sliced red onion, ½ cup drained canned mandarin orange sections, 1 crumbled slice bacon, and 2 tablespoons reduced-fat dressing
4 lean proteins	4 ounce grilled salmon
	water

Evening Snack

1 milk	Hot cocoa: 1 cup heated fat-free milk mixed with 1 to 2 rounded teaspoons cocoa powder and Splenda to taste

Real Life: Pizza

I don't want you to stop eating nearly everyone's favorite food, pizza. But the idea is to be more prudent about how many slices you eat at one time. If you are in Group 2 or 3, this would be the place in the day to add a second slice, especially if you lead a highly active lifestyle.

Real Life: Sausage

One of my Good Mood Diet Clubs added the Morningstar sausages at breakfast. They loved them for the taste, nutrition benefit (from its soy content), and the perceived "splurge of eating sausages" after a lifetime of thinking it was healthier to avoid them.

Day 10

Breakfast

1 bread, 1 medium-fat protein	1 slice whole-wheat toast with 1 poached egg
1 milk, 1 fruit, 1 fat	1 cup fat-free sugar-free yogurt with 1 sliced banana or ¾ cup blueberries and 1 tablespoon ground flaxseed
	water

Morning Snack

1 milk, 2 very lean proteins	Homemade smoothie: Blend until smooth 1 cup fat-free milk, 14 grams of protein from flavored isolated whey protein powder, and 3 ice cubes

Lunch

1 bread	½ cup brown rice
2 vegetables, 3 very lean proteins, 1 fat	Shrimp stir-fry: 1 cup Chinese vegetables, 3 ounces shrimp, onion, garlic, and ginger stir-fried in 1 teaspoon peanut oil
	water

Afternoon Snack

1 fruit	½ cup dried mango
1 vegetable	½ cup vegetable or tomato juice
1 fat	6 dry-roasted almonds
	water

Dinner

1 bread	1 cup roasted potatoes and parsnips
1 bread, 1 fat	1 slice hearty whole-grain bread with 1 teaspoon Smart Balance Omega-3 spread
2 vegetables	1 cup roasted carrots, onions, and garlic
4 lean proteins	4 ounces roasted dark-meat turkey or chicken
1 fat	8 black olives
1 fruit	1 Metropolitan (page 203)

Evening Snack

1 milk	Hot cocoa: 1 cup heated fat-free milk mixed with 1 to 2 rounded teaspoons cocoa powder and Splenda to taste

Real Life: Stir-Fries

Real Life: Asian food — especially stir-fries — is a terrific way to include onions, garlic, and ginger in your diet. People who eat a lot of onion and garlic have lower rates of gastrointestinal tract cancers, such as stomach and colon cancer. Ginger may also help to decrease migraine and arthritis pain, diminish risk of blood clots, and lower blood cholesterol levels.

Real Life: Olives

Add those healthy-fat olives to your diet! My favorite olives are from Kalamata, Greece. Olives and extra-virgin olive oil are rich in brain-cell building and abdominal fat-burning healthy fats.

Day 11

Breakfast

1 bread, 1 fat	½ cup cooked oats (not instant) with 1 tablespoon ground flaxseed and Splenda to taste
1 fruit	1¼ cups whole strawberries, sliced (or 1 diced apple if berries are out of season)
1 milk	1 cup fat-free milk
1 medium-fat protein	1 egg (cooked any way without fat)
	water

Morning Snack

1 milk, 2 very lean proteins	Homemade smoothie: Blend until smooth 1 cup fat-free milk, 14 grams of protein from flavored isolated whey protein powder, and 3 ice cubes

Lunch

1 bread	1 cup tomato soup
2 vegetables, 1 fat	2 cups mixed green salad with 2 tablespoons reduced-fat olive oil and balsamic vinegar dressing
3 very lean proteins	3 ounces turkey
	water

Afternoon Snack

1 fruit	8 dried apricot halves
1 vegetable	½ cup vegetable or tomato juice
1 fat	10 peanuts
	water

Dinner

2 bread,	2 salmon burritos: 2 (6-inch) whole-wheat tortillas
2 vegetables, 4 lean	rolled around 2 cups vegetables (shredded lettuce, red
proteins, 2 fats	cabbage, and tomato), 4 ounces grilled or broiled wild
	salmon, ⅛ sliced avocado, 3 tablespoons reduced-fat
	sour cream, and ½ cup salsa (free)
1 fruit	1 orange
	water

Evening Snack

1 milk	Hot cocoa: 1 cup heated fat-free milk mixed with 1 to
	2 rounded teaspoons cocoa powder and Splenda to
	taste

Real Life: Burritos

The favorite meal in my house is burritos. The kids love them because they're fun to put together (we all assemble our own from ingredients placed out on the table), fun to eat, and taste great. My husband and I love them because there's hardly any preparation or cleanup, and they get lots of good nutrition into all of us. Have fun!

Day 12

Breakfast

1 bread	1 slice whole-grain toast
1 fruit	1 medium banana
1 milk, 1 medium-fat protein, 1 fat	Mocha smoothie: Blend until smooth 1 cup fat-free milk, 4 ounces silken tofu, 1 tablespoon flaxseed meal, 1 cup strongly brewed coffee (free), 1 to 2 rounded teaspoons cocoa powder (free), Splenda to taste, and 2 to 3 ice cubes

Morning Snack

1 milk, 2 very lean proteins	Homemade smoothie: Blend until smooth 1 cup fat-free milk, 14 grams of protein from flavored isolated whey protein powder, and 3 ice cubes

Lunch

1 bread	1 cup chicken and vegetable noodle soup
2 vegetables, 1 fat	2 cups mixed green salad with 2 tablespoons reduced-fat olive oil and balsamic vinegar dressing
3 very lean proteins	3 ounces turkey
	water

Afternoon Snack

1 fruit	1 orange
1 vegetable, 1 fat	1 cup mini carrots with ½ tablespoon natural peanut butter
	water

Dinner

2 breads,	Turkey burger: 1 whole-wheat hamburger bun,
4 lean proteins,	4 ounces ground turkey patty, lettuce leaf, sliced
1 vegetable	tomato and onion, pickle, and 1 tablespoon ketchup
	and mustard (free)
1 vegetable, 1 fat	1 cup tossed salad with 2 tablespoons reduced-fat
	salad dressing
1 fat	8 black olives
1 fruit	1 Blackberry Bliss (page 199)
	water

Evening Snack

1 milk	Hot cocoa: 1 cup heated fat-free milk mixed with 1 to
	2 rounded teaspoons cocoa powder and Splenda to
	taste

Real Life: Soup

Soup is an important staple in the Good Mood Diet. It fills you up, provides fluid, and is packed with hearty nutrition. During the dark days of winter, there's nothing like a warm bowl of soup. And during the summer months, cool off with a cold gazpacho or fruit soup.

Day 13

Breakfast

1 bread, 1 medium-fat protein, 1 fat	Egg salad pita: ½ whole-wheat pita bread, stuffed with 1 chopped hard-boiled egg, 1 tablespoon ground flaxseed, and 2 tablespoons plain nonfat yogurt and 2 tablespoons salsa (free)
1 fruit	½ grapefruit
1 milk	1 cup fat-free milk
	water

Morning Snack

1 milk, 2 very lean proteins	Homemade smoothie: Blend until smooth 1 cup fat-free milk, 14 grams of protein from flavored isolated whey protein powder, and 3 ice cubes

Lunch

1 bread	½ medium or 1 small baked potato
3 very lean proteins, 1 fat	½ cup chili without beans
2 vegetables	2 cups tossed green salad, with 2 tablespoons fat-free dressing (free)
	water

Afternoon Snack

1 fruit	8 dried apricot halves
1 vegetable	½ cup vegetable or tomato juice
1 fat	1 tablespoon Tamari-roasted sunflower seeds
	water

Dinner

2 breads, 4 lean proteins, 2 fats, 1 fruit, 1 vegetable	2 fish tacos: 2 taco shells stuffed with 4 ounces cod (or other fish) sautéed in 2 teaspoons canola oil, ½ cup mango salsa, and 1 cup shredded red and green cabbage and onions
1 vegetable	1 cup tossed salad, with 2 tablespoons fat-free salad dressing (free)
	water

Evening Snack

1 milk	Hot cocoa: 1 cup heated fat-free milk mixed with 1 to 2 rounded teaspoons cocoa powder and Splenda to taste

Real Life: Eggs

Eggs are a potent nutritional package. Their protein is as high-quality as it comes. The yolk is full of lecithin, so important for memory and prevention of diseases of the brain. If your heart and blood vessels are healthy, there is no reason not to eat an egg every day. If not, lecithin is also found in soy, so you can alternate soy with the egg, or substitute a soy-based food for an egg to feed your brain and your body.

There are all kinds of ways of fixing eggs. The morning egg salad feels like such a treat but really isn't much work at all. One Good Mood Dieter added the ground flaxseed to the egg white omelet. She loved it!

Day 14

Breakfast

1 bread	1 slice whole-wheat toast
1 milk, 1 fruit, 1 fat	1 cup plain fat-free yogurt, mixed with 1 sliced banana or 1¼ cups fresh strawberries, 1 tablespoon ground flaxseed, and Splenda to taste
1 medium-fat protein	2 Morningstar Farm Veggie Breakfast Sausage Links
	water

Morning Snack

1 milk, 2 very lean proteins	Homemade smoothie: Blend until smooth 1 cup fat-free milk, 14 grams of protein from flavored isolated whey protein powder, and 3 ice cubes

Lunch

1 bread, 2 vegetables, 2 very lean proteins, 1 fat	1 cup Manhattan Clam Chowder (page 156)
1 very lean protein	Egg-white scramble: spray skillet with cooking spray and cook 2 beaten egg whites over medium heat
	water

Afternoon Snack

1 fruit	1 apple
1 vegetable	½ cup vegetable or tomato juice
1 fat	10 peanuts (ballpark-style take longer to eat!)
	water

Dinner

1 bread, 1 fat	1 large corn on cob rubbed with 1 teaspoon extra-virgin olive oil
1 bread, 1 fat	½ cup sweet potato, sprinkled with 1 tablespoon dry-roasted sunflower seeds
2 vegetables	1 cup steamed Brussels sprouts with spicy mustard (free)
4 lean proteins	4 ounces grilled or broiled lean meat (beef, pork, lamb, dark meat poultry)
1 fruit	1 orange
	water

Evening Snack

1 milk	Hot cocoa: 1 cup heated fat-free milk mixed with 1 to 2 rounded teaspoons cocoa powder and Splenda to taste

Real Life

This day's lunch can seem like a lot of food to some clients. But it will be the right sort of food to fuel your afternoon — rather than one that prompts you to take a nap. Meat is a mood booster in the right portions and this dinner adds other items and flavors to help you to become accustomed to meat being more side dish than prominent dish.

When it comes to nonstarchy vegetables like Brussels sprouts, cabbage, lettuce, peppers, and cucumbers, don't feel you have to limit your portions. The goal is to include at least five servings each day. So if you order, say, a large salad, don't sweat it if it's bigger than 2 cups. Enjoy it! It's good for you.

A Good Mood Breakthrough Story:

DON'T FORGET ABOUT CHOCOLATE MILK

As a member of the United States Olympic women's hockey team at the 2006 Winter Olympics in Turin, Italy, Kelly Stephens scored the first goal in the game that earned her team the Bronze Medal. She played on the top offensive lines and was praised for her energy by coaches and broadcasters alike.

A few months before the Games, Kelly wasn't feeling so great about her energy level on the ice. "Since I was sleeping relatively well and doing the same amount of exercise each day, I thought I should experiment with my eating habits," she recalls.

So she called her dad, who in turn called me. I promised both Kelly and her dad that working with me would be a full immersion into practical and realistic suggestions on what to eat and when.

Kelly emailed me after the Olympics to say how much she appreciated those "very practical" details. "I've found most nutritional advice to be extremely complex," she told my coauthor, Bob, during an interview. "I needed someone to tell me what foods that I liked were OK and when in my day to eat them to benefit the most. That is exactly what Susan was able to do. She gave me a practical plan, one that I could do while on the road and even at the Olympic Village."

My advice included "don't forget about chocolate milk" as a potential recovery drink after practice or games. A new study even backs up my shorthand sports nutrition.

Kelly wondered if pizza was nutritious and if it could fit into the Good Mood plan. I said, sure, but don't eat the food favorite for both lunch and dinner, because it could lead to feeling sluggish. For an optimal postgame meal, I suggested fish tacos with vegetables and rice, plus a large banana. Because of her highly active lifestyle — hockey shifts, or turns on the ice during a game, are typically a minute or two because the players go so hard — I recommended lemonade for the beverage.

I also talked to Kelly about becoming more proficient at fueling her muscles for optimal performance and, not to be overlooked, optimal recovery and rest. She was snacking on fresh fruit, for instance — a good idea. But I urged her to add low-fat mozzarella sticks and a handful of almonds. She fueled her Olympic run with her own personalized trail mix of dried fruits and nuts that she brought with her to Italy.

Kelly, like many Olympians, was regularly instructed to drink a sports drink before, during, and after practice. But she admits to not being disciplined about such timely consumption until we agreed it was a formal part of her plan. One key change for Kelly was always making sure to get the sports drink after the game or practice; it sets up the body for recovery and more zip the next day.

Plus, I added a V8 Juice and fruit yogurt in the hour before practice to fuel the body for longer-lasting energy. Kelly says she has noticed the difference and that she didn't experience the usual weight loss of several pounds or more after a game or hard practice. She felt less drained. "My energy levels were so much more even," Kelly says. "I could focus on playing well rather than whether I was tired."

4

THE GOOD MOOD KITCHEN

The key to making the Good Mood plan work is, well, the planning. Most of us don't take the time anymore — and many people don't even know how — to plan effectively. Planning was something that our grandmothers used to do, especially in the kitchen.

We're going to change that. You can establish a Good Mood kitchen in your life. And it won't take up a lot of extra time in your day. In fact, most of my clients enjoy the planning and even come to love it. They see it as a way to be in more control of their lives — no small matter if you ask a stress researcher.[1]

Few families have a designated nutrition planner these days. This is a person who thinks about the menus, makes the shopping list, goes to the supermarket, and makes the meals. It is a role that can be shared in a customized permutation, but just make sure the duties are clearly defined.

Most families fly by the seat of their pants, deciding what they'll eat just as they notice they're hungry. Fast food, boxed meals, and prepared foods rule. The result is nothing short of an anxious, undernourished, and overfed society.

My coauthor, Bob, would argue that the designated planner system works even in a house of college students. When he was in college, he and one of his seven roommates — both guys turned out to be health journalists, go figure — developed an egalitarian cooking schedule for the school year and assigned a pair of guys each week to shop for a standardized grocery list. The guys in the house were able to rely on hot breakfasts, portable lunches, and sit-down dinners. They were on their own for snacks, but, hey, it was the late 1970s and too early for the Good Mood strategies of mid-morning smoothies and mid-afternoon trail mixes. Not coincidentally, those college friends were successful students and have stayed close throughout life. There was a lot of friendship served up during those meals, along with the more practical brain and body fueling.

In order to achieve success in any part of life, you have to have a plan. It's hard to accomplish goals, short-term or long-term, without a plan. Most people who are financially stable have some kind of a financial plan, even if it is as simple as "don't spend money." People with career goals set a path to follow as they move through education and job settings. If you want to have health and fitness goals, you need a plan, too, and must follow through with it. All of these plans take a bit of attention on a regular basis to keep the plan on track.

We've done some of the planning work for you to ease your way into the Good Mood Diet. Start with the Good Mood Menus (page 64): Choose the meals that look best to you and plan out at least several days of meals. You can swap any lunch for any other lunch. The same with breakfasts and dinners, and morning and afternoon snacks. Or if you really love an entrée from one meal, you can repeat it even if it's not repeated in the menu.

Follow the Good Mood shopping list.

Now that you've got your meals planned, you can use our shopping list to check off the foods that you'll need to buy. The menus are based on the Feel-Great Foods; those are your staple foods. In little time, you'll just know what foods you need to stock in the Good Mood Kitchen.

In fact, this is a critical strategy: Make sure the food you need is on hand when you need it. You want to be prepared when you're hungry. That way you stick to your plan, rather than relying on whatever is around. The Feel-Great Foods become your fast and easy foods too.

The Good Mood Shopping List is detailed at the end of this chapter, starting on page 110.

Keep it simple in the Good Mood Kitchen.

You want this plan to work, and not be a burden. People always ask me if I spend hours in the kitchen. No way! I have two school-age children, I run my own business, and my husband operates his own business. Our family meals have to be easy and simple, or the food won't get on the table. The Good Mood goal is to make this as practical as possible.

That doesn't mean that if you like to spend time in the kitchen that this will be boring. We have created delicious recipes for you to have fun with and enjoy. Just follow the basic outline for the day's menus and then substitute the recipes that you like from Chapter 8. Even better, I'll teach you how to figure out how to include your own favorite recipes in the Good Mood Diet. Once you really understand what you are eating, just about any meal, snack, and favorite food fits.

How practical is that?

Just like learning anything new, it takes a little time to learn the basics. People who begin the Good Mood Diet say it takes them a week to ten days to get onto "cruise control" with the program. Some habits you will adopt practically overnight. In any case, it is a short timeframe to establish a lifelong plan that works for you and not the other way around.

At first you'll need to think about what you need to eat and when you need to eat it throughout the day. You will need to refer back to the template of how many servings of, say, bread, very lean protein, or medium-fat proteins are at each meal or snack. But it will come naturally soon enough.

The best strategy for learning your plan is to keep track of what you're eating. Whether you call it logging or journaling, writing down what you eat is the best way to turn old habits into new ones, and to learn the program itself.[2] Make copies of the Good Mood Log in Appendix B so that you can track how you're doing every day.

Once you know the daily plan, you'll realize that you are not thinking about it so much anymore. All of a sudden you'll notice that your habits have changed and you are reaching for Feel-Great Foods without thinking twice. It takes most of my clients no more than about ten days.

Equip your kitchen to facilitate Good Mood eating and planning.

Another strategy to make things easier is to have the right kinds of cooking utensils available in your kitchen. Here is a list of tools and gadgets that I really use in my kitchen:

Good Mood Cooking Supplies

- **A couple of good knives:** Every chef calls knives his or her greatest tools. Don't cheap out when buying the knives and be certain to have a reliable system for sharpening. We use ceramic sharpening stones and sharpen our blades after every couple of uses.
- **Blender:** Nothing fancy, but remember you will be chopping up ice for smoothies so it needs to be fairly powerful.
- **Covered shaker cup:** I use this when I need to take my smoothies on the road. Some containers can be frozen, which then thaws out during your commute. One of my Good Mood Diet Clubs discovered a portable smoothie jug that freezes in the middle so you have no sweating on the outside surface.
- **Foaming wand:** This is an electronic whisk that is marketed for making latte foam in thirty seconds or less. I use it to thoroughly mix cocoa (which is more dense in its pure form) into milk.
- **Food processor:** A smaller one is adequate and creates wonderful sauces and flavors with much less work than you might think.
- **Juicer:** I love mine and use it many times a week, although it is not necessary to the Good Mood plan.
- **Measuring cups and spoons:** Keep them in a handy place in your kitchen.

- **Two (small and large) nonstick fry pans, one with a cover:** If yours are worn, put it in your budget to get new ones.
- **Rice cooker:** This item is one of the underrated items in the Good Mood Kitchen. Easy to use, but make sure you buy one with a setting for brown rice.
- **Nonstick wok:** Changes the way you think about stir-fries because it simplifies preparation and cleanup while boosting flavor. Now, that's Good Mood cooking.
- **Nonstick broiler pan:** I use mine several times a week to prepare fish.
- **Rubber or plastic cooking utensils for use in nonstick pans:** To avoid those scratches. Pay attention to how the utensils feel in your hand.
- **Turkey cooking bags (large for whole turkey, small for turkey breast):** Simple and easy. Repeat, simple and easy.
- **Coffee grinder:** Buy whole coffee beans and grind enough for the day or a few days at most. I'm particular enough that I grind only what I need each time so that they stay as fresh as possible.
- **Very small coffee grinder:** I dedicate this item for grinding flaxseed.
- **Tea ball:** An optional item, if you prefer loose green tea rather than bags.
- **Electric can opener:** Optional, but great for canned tuna and beans.
- **Microwave-safe bowls:** For heating up leftovers. The idea is to make it smooth and effort-free to follow your plan.
- **Storable plastic containers with lids:** For leftovers or packing meals/snacks. Take the time to find a store with a good selection. Pick sizes and types that fit your household needs.
- **Good thermos:** I have two kinds, one for soups, one for drinks.
- **Insulated lunch carrier:** This can be optional but I find the thermal bag works for packing snacks and serves to remind me to plan ahead.
- **Ice packs:** to put in your insulated lunch carrier and keep cold foods cold, and safe.

Don't abandon your favorite recipe —
re-fit them for Good Mood.

How can you ever know if your favorite recipe fits into the Good Mood plan? It's easy. I'll teach you how I figure it out.

The menus are based on a certain number of bread, protein, milk, vegetable, fruit, and fat servings every day — as discussed in the Good Mood Template section of Chapter 3 (page 54). So when you look at a recipe, or a dish that's a combination of different ingredients, you just have to figure out how many servings of the different food groups are in one serving of that food.

You can simply "ballpark" what you're eating. If I would do that with pizza, I'd figure that a slice of pizza crust looks bigger than a slice of bread. So I would count it as 1½ slices. It would be hard to get more than one ounce of cheese on one slice, so there's the one protein serving. It's a high fat cheese, so I'd figure at least a medium-fat protein serving plus another fat serving. Then the tomato sauce and any added vegetables would be close to one vegetable serving, but not quite. That's pretty close, and can certainly work well enough as long as you don't eat pizza every day.

Let's look at some other favorite foods, such as a baked potato:

If it's a small potato, then it's considered one bread/starch serving. But that's a really small potato. Think about what would fit into ½ cup. So most baked potatoes, if you eat the whole potato, will likely be closer to two servings rather than one.

Did you put butter on your potato? One teaspoon is one fat serving. If you have a premade "pat" of butter, that's one serving.

What about cheese sauce? When you're out at a restaurant, figure that most of the sauce is fat, not protein, and count the sauce as two fat servings.

Next, let's estimate a bowl of soup: how about chicken noodle. One cup of chicken noodle soup will probably be about a third noodles. There's only a tiny bit of chicken in there, and while the rest of the soup is robust with cooked veggies, vitamins, and minerals, those get to come on board for free. Count 1 cup of chicken noodle soup as one bread/starch serving. If it's a big bowl, it's probably two servings. Split pea soup follows the same formula.

Bean soups are measured the same way, but remember that beans are a good source of protein and starch. So 1 cup of bean soup counts as one very lean protein and one starch serving. If it's a big bowl chock-full of beans, count it as two of each.

If you're eating a cream soup, there's got to be some fat in there. Add one to two fat servings per cup.

Chili varies from all beans to bean and meat to meat only. The meat is usually lean meat. In 1 cup there may be ⅓ to ½ cup of beans and about 1 ounce of meat. And then the tomato sauce, paste, and other ingredients make 1 cup of meat-and-bean chili about two lean meat servings and two starch servings. As your portion size increases, so do the number of servings. If you don't have any beans in your chili, or just a few, then drop one starch serving.

What about Asian food? Remember that ½ cup of cooked vegetables is one serving. So your standard Asian entrée is probably going to be at least 1 cup of vegetables, or two vegetable servings. You'll usually have about 2 ounces of protein per serving. If it's shellfish or white chicken, then that's very lean protein. If it's dark chicken, pork, or beef, figure lean protein. There's usually some kind of thickener/sweetener added, so add one starch serving. And then at least one fat serving. If it seems pretty oily to you, add another fat serving. Then figure in your noodles or rice. Every ½ cup is one bread/starch serving.

As for Sunday brunch, there are two approaches here. If this is a celebration or an infrequent affair, go ahead and enjoy yourself and don't worry about counting your servings. Eat what you most enjoy and don't bother with the mediocre offerings. If this is an every Sunday occurrence, then some diligence as to what you are eating may be in order.

All of these concepts apply wherever you go. Even at home. But when you're eating at a restaurant, unless it's highly unusual, figure that fat is added to everything you eat. So when you take a scoop of mashed potatoes, figure double the fat that you add at home. A ½ cup serving of restaurant mashed potatoes will have one bread/starch serving plus one fat serving. Noodles and rice will fall into the same category.

Egg dishes have one whole egg (a medium-fat protein) in every ½ cup serving. Always add one fat serving and then whatever else you see. Does it have cheese? Add another medium-fat protein plus another fat serving.

Look at the pancakes and waffles. Are they the size of a slice of bread or really more like two slices? The same goes for bagels. Is it a small, frozen-style bagel where half a bagel equals one slice of bread, or are they large bagels where each bagel half is more like one and a half slices of bread?

Develop an awareness of your supermarket route up and down the aisles: Stick to the perimeter.

If you were in one of my Good Mood Diet Clubs in Seattle, Chicago, Cleveland, or other cities you'd attend the second group meeting at a local supermarket. Learning how to shop is a big part of making this program as easy as it is effective. So I'm going to take you on a cart's-eye tour of a supermarket to help you streamline your shopping trips to your local store.

Imagine that you have entered the front doors of your supermarket. Looking straight ahead you probably see rows and rows of boxed and bottled products. If you look all the way to your right, all the way to your left, and all the way to the back of the store, you'll see the foods that usually don't come in boxes. These are the most natural foods, found all along the outside walls of the store.

Do most of your shopping on the perimeter of the store; that's where you'll find the produce, butcher, fishmonger, dairy case, and fresh bakery. The closer you get to the middle of the store, the more processed the food.

Paula Burke and Jennifer Lail, two of the group members featured in the *Seattle Post-Intelligencer* columns that helped inspire this book, met at the newspaper's offices for a one-year update photo. They lingered after the photo session to trade notes on their first twelve months on the Good Mood plan. Both agreed on the single-best habit learned. It was "sticking to that perimeter of the store," said Paula. "It changed everything for me," added Jennifer.

You should know that foods are placed on the shelves of the store with a very specific strategy. Food manufacturers pay for their placements in the supermarket — on shelves, in the dairy case, along the bread racks, you name it. The more the company pays, the closer to eye level its product will be placed. Where a product is located on the shelf is no indication of how good it is for you. And very often the Feel-Great products are on the bottom shelves.

There is one exception. That's in stores that have specific aisles devoted to "health" foods. You might well see Good Mood cereals at eye level or organic soups higher than your knees. But keep in mind that even here some so-called healthy foods are highly processed and not great choices for Good Mood eating. And those companies are still paying for their premium shelf space.

Back to the all-important perimeter of the store. Let's start at the produce section, usually the most visually pleasing area of the store. Notice the variety of colors and shapes. Try to shop keeping such variety in mind. It is strategic not only to eat a variety of foods among the food groups, but also a range of foods within each food group. Along with broccoli from the brassica vegetable group (and the suggested at least one daily serving), eat cabbage, cauliflower, Brussels sprouts, and bok choy. Along with lettuce, eat spinach, kale, and Swiss chard. A sweet potato is just as easy to microwave as a white potato.

Fruit follows the same concept. While apples and bananas are terrific staples for your fruit bowl, broaden your shopping list with whatever is in season and looks best: oranges, grapefruit, pomegranates, peaches, nectarines, plums, berries, cherries, grapes. All have different levels of vitamins, minerals, phytochemicals, and food factors that will keep you healthy and make you feel good. For berries, you can keep up the daily-serving recommendation by going to frozen bags that easily thaw.

Always choose the fruits and vegetables that look the freshest. If you're shopping for a recipe that calls for leaf lettuce, but the leaf lettuce looks terrible that day, don't buy it. Substitute something else, or switch to another recipe. Get to know the produce manager and don't hesitate to ask whether he's got some better-looking tomatoes in the back. Pleasing customers is the produce manager's business.

The produce section is usually where you'll find products like tofu, freshly packed nuts, and dried fruits, plus 100-percent juices that need to be refrigerated. These are all good choices to include in your shopping cart.

Go organic when possible for the Earth, the farm workers, and our children.

Many supermarkets now have an organic produce section. I am an advocate of organic produce because I think it is a better form of sustainable agriculture for the Earth. There is fairly good evidence that farm workers who apply chemicals to crops have a high rate of chemical contamination in their bodies, which is linked to increased risks of cancer. In addition, there is some data showing children who eat organically grown produce have a significantly lower urinary output of chemical metabolites compared with children eating a diet of conventionally grown produce.[3]

There is less data about the nutritional content of organic produce. A few small studies have shown better nutrition profiles in organic produce versus conventionally grown produce, but this difference is unremarkable at this point.[4] Some people claim that organic produce tastes better. There is even something called the Brix that grades sugar content, amino acids, oils, flavonoids, minerals, and other nutrients in produce; organic fruits and veggies often get higher Brix scores than conventional produce.[5] Bottom line: In many cases I agree with the argument that organic tastes better.

On the other hand, organic produce is often more expensive than conventionally grown produce. When weighing the risks and benefits of how you spend your food dollars, the current data are quite clear: We know populations that don't eat fruits and vegetables are not as healthy as those with diets abundant in fruits and vegetables, regardless of the application of chemicals to the crops. We have no similar comparison between organic and conventionally grown produce. So if your choice is conventionally grown produce or none at all, do not let any fears stop you from buying fresh, delicious, conventionally grown produce. But don't be afraid to ask produce managers about the sources of their wares and make trips to local farmers' markets (where you can quiz growers directly about pesticides).

If cost is not an impediment, then go organic. It is better for the Earth, and there is no question that it is better for the farm workers. Lots of parents are convinced it is healthier and safer for their children. You might find that it tastes a little better. By voting with our wallets, we can all influence the market enough to make it a highly profitable agricultural strategy, increasing the production and bringing down the price to make it available to all.

As you leave the produce section at the supermarket, you next usually find the butcher and fishmonger. Here again, think variety: chicken, turkey, lamb, lean beef, lean pork, and all the different kinds of fish and shellfish. Buy some for now, and buy some to put in the freezer so that you always have options available. Remember that serving sizes for the Good Mood Menus are typically 3 to 4 ounces.

The organic question comes into play with meat, and also with milk products. Because so many of the contaminants in food are fat soluble, and meat and dairy products are a source of fat in our diets, I always prefer organic, whenever possible. It reduces the amount of antibiotic residue that we are consuming, which is a good strategy for future health.

And you may find that organic meats taste better. This is not an absolute, but often the case. If you must choose between organic and conventional for financial reasons, or if organic isn't available to you, then choose the freshest meat and milk products available, and enjoy them.

On to the dairy case. Here you have many choices beyond the organic. First, choose nonfat or low-fat milk products. You easily reduce fat and cholesterol intake by using these products, and leave room for more fat servings the rest of the day.

One of the deep concerns about milk is many people suffer from the inability to digest lactose, the sugar naturally found in milk. While many people lose their ability to digest a lot of lactose at one time as they age, most people still have some small capability to digest lactose. Clients I have counseled report previous sinus and congestive reactions to dairy, especially milk.

Here's my answer and it almost always plays out successfully, whether dairy reluctance is digestive or sinus-related. Avoid discomfort by consuming only 1 cup (8 ounces) maximum at a time, just as I've designed in the menus.

Many people can also eat yogurt and cheese, even when milk gives them discomfort. And goat milk is lower in lactose than cow's milk, so you can always give that a try.

Beware the added sugar in processed foods, even in health-food yogurt.

Yogurt will be in this dairy section too. I am a big fan of yogurt. The bacterial cultures, called probiotics, are so helpful in maintaining gut health, i.e., keeping the diseases and discomforts of the intestines at bay. However, the food industry has taken one of man's best joint efforts with nature and moved it toward the junk-food pile.

Look on the side of an average 6-ounce carton of yogurt and you'll find the nutrition facts label. A low-fat yogurt will have somewhere around 2.5 grams of total fat. Nonfat varieties have less or none. Most yogurts will have 7 to 9 grams of protein. All are good numbers and within the Good Mood template. It's the amount of sugar that bends and spindles the Good Mood parameters. It can be downright upsetting to individuals who are watching how much added sugar is in their diet. Trust me, I have seen numerous clients walk away with heads shaking in frustration after checking yogurt labels. "I thought I was doing such a good thing for myself," is a typical comment.

Let's dissect the sugar content so that you have a factual basis for comparing one yogurt product to the next.

Milk contains a total of 12 grams of carbohydrates per cup. All of the carbohydrates come from milk sugar, known as lactose. When you read the side of a 6- to 8-ounce carton of plain, unsweetened yogurt, you will see that it contains 12 to 15 grams of carbohydrates, and 12 to 15 grams of sugar. (Ranges are given because different yogurts are more or less watery, so the amount of space left for solids differs.) This is what is naturally found in milk. Nothing is added to the yogurt. When you purchase any plain, nonfat yogurt, there may be a little bit of extra carbohydrates added if you find thickening agents in the ingredients list. But there won't be any more sugar in 8 ounces than 12 to 15 grams. However, once you select flavored yogurts with sweeteners, the amount of sugar can range from 12 grams to more than 30. Any amount of sugar above 12 to 15 grams is added to the product.

For instance, a carton of low-fat vanilla yogurt contains 25 grams of sugar. Twelve grams are found naturally in the milk, so 13 grams of sugar are added to the yogurt. One teaspoon of sugar is 4 grams, so there is a little more than 3 teaspoons of sugar added to this carton of yogurt. And this one is light on the added sugar.

Do you want to spend almost four of your 6 extra teaspoons of added sugar twice each week on one carton of yogurt? There are more brands with even more sugar added. But now you can figure out exactly how much is added, and how much was added by Mother Nature.

My choice and recommendation is to buy plain yogurt and add your own fruit and, if you need it, a sweetener such as a drizzle of maple syrup. The yogurt tastes fresher, and I know it will make you feel great all day long. Plus, you can save the added teaspoons of sugar for a dessert.

Learn the easy choices, then work on ways to fit favorite foods into the Good Mood plan.

Most of the clients that I take through the supermarket are very eager to get to the cheese section and find out whether they can still eat their favorite kind. Here's what I teach them:

Start with the easy choices.

Mozzarella cheese sticks weigh just about 1 ounce each. They contain 8 grams of protein and 2 to 5 grams of fat. At 2 grams of fat, one cheese stick is equivalent to one lean protein serving. At 5 grams of fat, one stick is equivalent to a medium-fat serving. Or you can count the same cheese stick as one very lean protein and one fat serving.

A great spreadable cheese is Laughing Cow Light Original Swiss. Each wedge contains 2.5 grams of protein and 2 grams of fat. You can eat three of these wedges and count it as one very lean protein serving plus one fat serving. This is a treat on whole-wheat crackers. You might even love to dip whole-wheat pretzels into the cheese.

Now you should be getting the picture of how to figure out how to include just about anything in your diet. Once you know what's really in the food, you just fit it into the menu plan. That's what I do for my clients, and even for myself.

Let's look at a more traditional cheese: Cheddar, for example. Just like all cheeses, 1 ounce is still 7 grams of protein, making it one protein serving. It's the fat that changes. Cheddar cheese has 9 to 10 grams of fat per ounce. One Good Mood fat serving is five grams. So the easiest way to count it is one very lean protein serving plus two fats. You can see that you'll need to enjoy smaller portions of higher-fat cheeses if you want to stay within the Good Mood guidelines.

On the other hand, if you are at a party and you don't usually eat cheese, go ahead and enjoy the assortment of lovely cheeses that are often at celebrations. Then remember to eat all the foods that you still need to eat that day. Tomorrow you'll be back on your Good Mood Menus and won't even notice a bump in the road.

Eggs are often positioned near the dairy case. These days, there are quite a number of choices. The Good Mood Menus are based on large-sized eggs. Then there are the choices of vegetarian-fed, free-range, omega-3–enhanced, and more. For all the same reasons as I stated above regarding meat and dairy, I like organic, vegetarian-fed the best. Omega-3–enhanced eggs are another useful way to supplement your diet with alpha-linolenic acid. The chickens are fed flaxseed to enhance omega-3 production. Often these eggs have a slightly lower cholesterol level.

Against the fourth wall of the supermarket you'll usually find the fresh bakery. Many upscale supermarkets have begun to include hearth-baked crusty breads as part of their selections. These fresh breads are very tasty and often have healthy ingredients like olives and nuts added. While there may be some whole-grain varieties, most are usually only partly whole-grain, or not at all. I like to balance the refined flours in these breads by dipping them in a teaspoon of delicious olive oil and rich balsamic vinegar.

Many bread makers are trying to capitalize on the benefits of flaxseed. But the flaxseed is usually added whole, not ground. You'll be able to see the seeds in the bread. Don't fall for this gimmick and pay extra for flax bread: There are no benefits to eating whole flaxseeds. They must be ground to gain the nutritional benefits.

As you begin to wind your way into the inner aisles of the supermarket, you can still find some Feel-Great foods. Going to the frozen section, you can stock up on frozen fruits to add to your smoothies. Purchase frozen fruits only without added syrups or sugars.

Frozen vegetables are valuable to have on hand. If you're a once-a-week shopper, or even less, frozen fruits and vegetables are a lifesaver. The vegetables in your freezer will be far more nutritious when compared to those that you bought a week ago and have wilted in the bottom of your refrigerator. Always look for varieties without added sauces.

Another plus in the freezer section: the Morningstar Farms soy sausage products that work in the Good Mood Plan. Discovered by one of my Good Mood Diet Club members, two of these sausage links add up to one medium-fat protein and work perfectly at breakfast. They are a nutritious breakfast protein alternative to an egg.

Not far from the frozen foods is the cereal aisle. This is where it becomes very clear what most of America is eating. The cereals with the least sugar added are usually down by your feet; those that are called *candy* in my house are right at eye level.

Using the same concept that we used to figure out how much sugar is added to yogurt, here is how you can figure out how much sugar is added to cereal. First, pick up a box of shredded wheat and find the nutrition facts label. You'll see that there is zero grams of sugar in shredded wheat. Grains do not naturally contain sugar. So *any* sugar listed on the label of a box of cereal is added sugar. The only exception is if there is fruit added to the cereal. Some small amount of the sugar (since very little fruit is really added) will come from added fruit. Remember, every 4 grams of sugar is equivalent to another teaspoon.

Next in the cereal decision, think fiber and protein. If you look back at that box of shredded wheat, you'll see that one serving (1 cup) contains 6 grams of fiber and 6 grams of protein. In the Good Mood Diet, one serving is ½ cup, but that still gives you 3 grams of fiber and 3 grams of protein; a very dense package of nutrition for relatively few calories. Use these values to compare other cereals that you pick up from the shelf. The mystery of which cereals are the least processed will be solved, and the results of highly processed food manufacturing will become quite clear.

Plus, you will get to eat cereal for breakfast again after too many years of the carbohydrate police and carb scares.

Use the least processed foods as your gold standards.

This strategy of comparing the nutritional content of the least processed food with others in the same category is one of the best ways I know to read labels and make choices in the supermarket. It gives you a standard by which you can compare one product to another. You might still choose a more processed product, but at least you'll know what you are eating.

To me, making an informed choice makes all the difference. Then you are choosing from knowledge rather than by default. That fact alone can make you feel good.

Those are the highlights of the Good Mood Supermarket Tour. Whether you are in the cereal aisle or the snack-food aisle, the principles stay the same. Check out all your favorite foods, or even new ones that you spot at the store, and see how they figure into your Good Mood Diet plan.

You can work around allergies and intolerance to fish, milk, and nuts.

If you are allergic to fish, you just can't eat it. If you can eat shellfish but not fish, or vice versa, then you are in luck. But if you can't eat either, then it is very important that you ask your physician about using an omega-3 nutritional supplement. Be careful that whatever you use will not cause allergic reactions. Ask your physician about marine algae oils and other vegetarian options.

If you are lactose intolerant, then you might still be able to drink small portions of milk, and eat yogurt, as mentioned above. By drinking only 1 cup of milk at a time, and mixing it with other foods, you may find that you don't experience the symptoms that you have in the past. If you are allergic to milk protein, then you need to avoid both the milk products and the whey protein supplement. In that case, use a soy supplement. You can use soy milk as a substitute for cow's milk. Purchase one that is fortified with calcium and vitamins A and D. Another option may be goat's milk. Rice milk is not a good substitute for cow's milk.

If you are allergic to nuts, then you must not eat the nuts in the menu plan. Substitute other healthy fats from avocados, olives, olive oil, and seeds.

For a detailed guide to added sugars in common processed foods, see Appendix C.

The Good Mood Shopping List

As promised, here's the shopping list that we've put together for the Good Mood Diet Club members and other clients that I've worked with. The club members say it makes starting the program much easier.

Fruits

Berries (fresh or frozen)

Citrus (fresh or juice)

Dried fruit (raisins, apricots, etc.)

Other fruit (mango, apples, pineapple, bananas, etc.)

Vegetables

Broccoli, cauliflower, Brussels sprouts, kohlrabi, cabbage

Carrots, mini carrots, sweet potatoes/yams, winter squash

Lettuce, spinach, kale, Swiss chard

Tomatoes, red and green sweet peppers

Onions, garlic, leeks

Other vegetables (green beans, okra, cucumbers, etc.)

Vegetable juice

Vegetable soups

Proteins

Turkey (fresh breast, deli-sliced, ground)

Chicken (light and dark meat; pieces or whole)

Fish (fresh, canned, or frozen)

Shellfish (fresh or frozen)

Lean meats (beef, pork, lamb, game)

Eggs, pasteurized egg whites

Beans (canned, frozen, dried)

Morningstar Farms Veggie Breakfast Sausage Links

Soy Crisps (in the healthy snack-food aisle)

Grains

Whole-grain breads

Whole-grain cereals (shredded wheat, oatmeal, Kashi, etc.)

Taco shells

Whole-wheat tortillas

Whole-grain buns, bagels

Brown rice (quick-cooking or regular)

Other grains (barley, buckwheat, etc.)

Dairy

Fat-free or low-fat milk

Fat-free or low-fat, sugar-free yogurt

Low-fat sour cream

Parmesan cheese

Low-fat mozzarella string cheese

Nuts and Seeds

Peanut butter or other nut butters (unsweetened)

Nuts (almonds, peanuts, etc.)

Whole or ground flaxseed

Fats and Oils

Olives

Olive oil

Canola oil

Peanut oil

Olive oil and balsamic vinegar salad dressing (regular or reduced-fat)

Condiments

Fat-free salad dressing

Mustard

Salsa

Balsamic vinegar

Raspberry vinegar

Non-dutched, no-alkali cocoa powder

Splenda

Spices

Sea salt or kosher salt

Black pepper

Cinnamon

Paprika

Ginger

Garlic

Turmeric

Supplements

Isolated whey protein powder

100% Daily Value multi-vitamin mineral supplement

Fish oil, omega-3 supplement (if desired)

Notes on Foods on the Shopping List

Cocoa

The phytochemicals found in natural, unprocessed cocoa beans are positive for lifting mood and lowering blood pressure. But the key is keeping the cocoa powders potent with those phytochemicals after they've been processed on the way from the rain forests to your supermarket.

Dutched cocoa powders are processed with alkalis to remove the bitterness from average cocoa beans. One major problem with that: The dutching process removes the important Feel-Great phytochemicals. High-quality cocoa beans processed with care but without alkali still have a smooth chocolate taste without the bitterness. Your goal is to find "natural," non-dutched cocoa powder. There are several options.

Hershey's "natural" cocoa powder is an inexpensive non-dutched product that is now available in many supermarkets.

Cocoa beans are now going the way of coffee beans. You can find organic, fair trade chocolates and cocoa powder, just the way that many coffee growers are now supported by fair trade practices. The majority of cocoa beans grown in the world come from the Ivory Coast in Africa. Many large-scale growers use slave labor and even child slave labor to work the fields. Fair trade practices ensure that growers are paid a fair price for their beans, thereby eliminating the need for slave or very low wage laborers so that they can make a profit.

While the cost of these fair trade products may be slightly higher, in my mind the price is well worth the social benefit. They are usually organic products, and you may find that they taste a little better, if only for the strife that you eliminate from the world. I know that I feel better in many ways because I purchase fair trade cocoa powder.

Dagoba Organic Cacao is a fair trade cocoa that is naturally processed. It is available at many specialty supermarkets like Whole Foods.

The best way to mix your delicious cocoa is to take a little bit of milk (a couple of tablespoons) and pour it into the bottom of your cup. Add the cocoa and make a paste. Then heat the rest of the milk in the microwave and mix it into the cocoa paste. Add Splenda if you desire and mix again. If you like, for a little fun you can whip the cocoa into a foam using one of those small hand-held battery-operated cappuccino whisks or foaming wands.

Fish and Safety

There are some safety issues with fish that otherwise fit the Good Mood profile. Large, predatory fish in our oceans may be contaminated with mercury. While the jury is still out on whether or not this mercury actually is biologically available in our bodies, if the answer turns out to be yes, it's enough mercury to be unsafe for health.[6] The fish that are most affected are swordfish, shark, and large tuna. If you eat these, limit your servings to just once a week.

While limiting swordfish and shark may not be difficult, limiting canned tuna can put the brakes on increasing your fish consumption. Worry not, I have a solution. Living in the Pacific Northwest, I am close to the docks for some of the country's busiest fishing vessels. One of these ships, Fishing Vessel St. Jude, fishes and cans small sized tuna (7 to 12 pounds) that contain no more mercury than any other living thing. Captain Joe Malley tests his catch each season for mercury content and it is certified to be at very safe levels.

Another reason to check out the kind of canned tuna from the boutique canneries of the Pacific Northwest is that the omega-3 fat content is many times higher in this tuna compared to tuna canned by the large commercial fishing giants like Starkist and Bumble Bee. These enormous fleets catch very large fish that are high in mercury, and then before canning they extract the wonderful oils rich in omega-3 fats and throw them overboard! Check the nutrition label on one of their cans and you'll find only ½ gram of fat per 2-ounce serving. Joe Malley's tuna contains 7 ounces of Feel-Great fats in each 2-ounce serving.

Try a can from either Fishing Vessel St. Jude (www.tunatuna.com) or Cinda's Sea Maiden's Harvest (www.seamaiden.com), and you won't be sorry. While their products are more expensive than the large commercial brands, you can be sure that you get what you pay for, plus peace of mind as well.

Whey Protein

As a sports nutritionist, I know that research — and my experience with clients — shows that whey protein is a great promoter of muscle recovery and growth before and after exercise. You get a double benefit from whey because it's also high in tryptophan, helping to keep your brain serotonin levels high. The Good Mood Diet has a targeted strategy for whey protein: Use it in your smoothie just after exercise, or at mid-morning as a regular snack, and you'll stay strong in mind and body all day long. Be sure to buy *isolated* whey protein so you have protein in its pure form without carbs or fats.

Omega-3 Supplements

You know that I always recommend food first. There is no replacement or substitute for the wonderful, natural sources of the hundreds of thousands of chemicals in food that we call nutrients, phytochemicals, and food factors. Supplements are just that, supplements to a good diet. But when it comes to omega-3 fats, the lines are not so black and white.

The omega-3 fats that our bodies use in greatest amounts are EPA and DHA. These fats come from marine oils, in other words, food from the sea. Found mostly in fish, they can also be found in small amounts in sea vegetables.

ALA, another omega-3 fat that is used in the body in small amounts and can also be transformed in the body into EPA and DHA, comes from land-based plant foods like flaxseed, cold-pressed vegetable oils, nuts, seeds, and some vegetables. While the body has the ability to transform ALA into EPA and DHA, it only has the capacity to transform 5 percent of the ALA into the other two forms, at the most. So while ALA is a nice supplement to a diet rich in omega-3 fats, it cannot substitute for them.

If you are not a fish eater, and are not going to eat fish no matter what I say in this book, then I encourage you to use omega-3 supplements. These fats are simply that critical to health and emotional well-being and that integral to the Good Mood strategy. I recommend supplementation on a daily basis to people who are not eating five fish meals each week.

There are many products on the market. These are the ones I like, and why:

Fisol: An enteric-coated DHA and EPA supplement containing 500 milligrams fish oil with 150 milligrams EPA and 100 milligrams DHA. The enteric coating allows digestion to occur in the intestines rather than in the stomach. Not only do you not have to contend with burping up fish oil, but absorption is improved as well. I take these with me when I travel, in case I can't get a good fish meal. It is available at many drug stores and online pharmacies.

Omega-3 Brain Booster: A powdered form of fish oil that has no odor and no taste. The oil is "coated" by a rice protein layer, making it ideal for those who can't swallow pills. It works great mixed into a smoothie or yogurt. Great for kids, but I periodically mix it into my post-workout smoothie when I know I'm not getting my five fish meals a week. It is available only online at www.omega3brainbooster.com.

If you are a vegetarian, it becomes especially difficult to get in enough omega-3s. There are a few DHA supplements that are derived from marine algae and encapsulated in nongelatin capsules. Search on the Internet for "algae oil" and you should find at least one or two products. The one that I am familiar with is made by Deva Nutrition.

You can imagine that a lot of research is going into how to produce an omega-3 fat supplement that is odorless and tasteless, and can be added to foods to fortify our food supply with these all-important fats.

Flaxseed

I mentioned that flaxseed is a nice supplement to a diet rich in EPA and DHA. Flaxseed is a potent source of alpha-linolenic acid (ALA), an essential fatty acid. Our bodies use ALA as is, without turning it into the other two omega-3 fats. Many people supplement with flaxseed oil. But most people consume enough ALA in their diets. In fact, there is some data that too much ALA may increase the risk of prostate cancer. I like ground seeds versus oil because, along with just a limited amount of the healthy fat, you get a very important fiber, lignin, which is found only in small amounts in our diets. Lignin is an indigestible fiber that may help control weight, blood sugar levels, and blood cholesterol. Additionally, lignins may actually help prevent prostate cancer. So I am an advocate of using ground flaxseed, and I do not recommend using flaxseed oil except occasionally.

You can buy flaxseed whole or already ground in a meal form. I prefer the seeds to flax oil. Always keep the seeds refrigerated or they will become rancid. The seeds must be ground for you to get the nutritional benefit. While cows have the kind of teeth and digestive system to chew up flaxseed, we don't, so the seeds come out the way they went in: whole. We must grind them first.

I like the taste best when freshly ground, so I have a tiny little burr coffee grinder at home that I use only for flax. I keep the seeds in the fridge and every morning I grind them and put them on my cereal. But I have ground flax meal around for when I travel. You'll read about that in the next chapter.

Good Mood Breakthrough Story:

NOBODY'S PERFECT — OR HAS TO BE

For Linda Behlke, one of the best things about the Good Mood Diet is not feeling like she has to be perfect.

"Dr. Kleiner made it clear from the start of our diet club, nobody is going to be perfect," says Linda. "Every other diet I have tried — and I have tried them all — you feel like either you do it perfectly or you are a failure."

Here's an important point. If you don't quite follow the Good Mood Menus some days, don't sweat it — but do your best to still eat the Good Mood foods such as one egg, your daily serving of flaxseed meal, the whey protein shake, and a hot cocoa before bed. You will still be doing something positive even on the most stressful days.

Linda lost 12 pounds in her first three months of the Good Mood plan — and that was during the winter holidays season. She especially likes "shrinking" into clothes that were too small just weeks ago.

"Things are going GREAT!" says Linda. "I'm amazed that I don't have any cravings and it seems painless to follow the program — I'm not tempted to overeat or indulge."

Linda has special reason to appreciate the Good Mood Plan. She has multiple sclerosis. "It can cause major fatigue," Linda says. "With Dr. Kleiner's plan, I have so much more energy and hope."

And fewer pounds.

5

THE GOOD MOOD TRAVELER

I t's time to get this Good Mood show on the road. Lots of diets work in the short-term for people, but then they reenter the atmosphere of reality. Many dieters go out into their days, live their lives, and typically fail to bring the diet along in the rumble seat.

You can break that flameout pattern with the Good Mood Diet. It has been fire-tested by hundreds of clients (and, frankly, me too) as they filled roles of workers, spouses, parents, adult children, aunts, uncles, friends, neighbors, community members, volunteers — you name it. All that life can sabotage most diets sooner or later. My intent for Good Mood readers is to always be a companion in feeling great, at home or anywhere you go.

We can all be Good Mood Travelers. Whether your "trip" is a daily commute, taking planes for your job or, aaahh, going on vacation, there is always room for improving your mood. It heightens every experience and fuels better performance. This chapter will highlight ways to stay in Good Mood territory no matter where your plans take you.

Scout your route.

In the last chapter we discussed how to navigate your local supermarket. I advise clients to do a similar canvas of their usual routes. We tend to be creatures of habit, going the same way to work or school. Whether it is your walk to the bus, the drive you make to work or the health club, the retail loop in your neighborhood, or a regular outing to see family, it is a Good Mood move to be aware of places that support your eating plan.

For instance, some of my clients can tell me exactly where they can buy a single hard-boiled egg in the morning or where they can find a coffeehouse that uses hormone-free milk. Others know the best places to find a Good Mood lunch or pick up some bulk almonds and dried fruit.

Finding a smoothie store isn't hard these days. But finding one that will make your mid-morning shake without added sugar can be harder. Don't hesitate to ask what brand of milk the smoothie shop uses or the type of protein powder. Look for one with whey protein.

I also keep an eye out for cafés with a respect for green tea, offering a few choices. It broadens my appreciation for the energizing drink, plus the right place offers an opportunity for the periodic ritual of catching up with myself over a steaming cup of tea. Or maybe I use that spot to meet a good friend.

Scouting your route is part of Good Mood planning. Some people like to keep actual notes on good spots, especially in work districts and down-town areas, then pass on the recommendations to other Good Mood Diet Club members. Others keep a mental list of what works for them. I say keep a page of good places in your daily planner notebook. The process of scouting and writing it down confirms your Good Mood strategies. Be a good scout for yourself.

Pack your meals and snacks when it is convenient.

First of all, this suggestion is a lot less work than it seems. Second, neglecting to pack on a certain day will not doom you to crankiness or poor performance. More about that in the next section of this chapter.

One of my secrets to packing is in my car. That's where I keep a regular stash of snacks — nuts, dried fruit, a case of water, some small vegetable juice cans. That way, if I dash out to pick up a child or make an appointment, I don't need to stop for snack packing. My kids and even some friends know that I am the healthy snack lady.

An important note about food in the car: That's where I stash it, but I don't suggest eating your snacks or lunch in the car. Find a place to stop, rest, and savor your food. Staying aware of what you eat doubles as both a way to better enjoy your food and a way to avoid overeating. It's difficult to taste food when you're fighting through traffic or making sure you follow the rules of the road.

What's more, no doubt you have read or heard about the statistics reporting that foods and drinks cause the most accidents. Hot coffee tops the list. I am not saying to never enjoy a latte in the car, but simply to ask if you are truly enjoying it that way. Carrying a water bottle for driving is safer and even serves to help curb hunger that is actually thirst. I keep a case of bottled water in my trunk (not in hot weather, it tastes terrible warm) to make it even easier to drink water during the day and on the go.

Another successful strategy is establishing a thermal lunch bag as part of your daily "luggage." You can clean it at night, then repack any dry, room-temperature items. I suggest putting it on the kitchen counter for easy packing of hot, cold, and perishable foods in the morning. I use one Thermos for hot soups and another for cold or hot drinks. Some thermal bags can hold two insulated containers plus still have room for your turkey sandwich, hard-boiled egg (if you are running late), carrot sticks with low-fat dip, and more.

Some Good Mood Diet Club members have purchased containers specifically to carry along the mid-morning smoothie. These particular containers have a core that fills with water to freeze, then keeps the drink cold until you consume it. I myself use an old-fashioned shaker to mix my mid-morning pick-me-up.

The vessel is less important than the habit. Find a way to keep drinking that smoothie, home or away, and your mood will be more even and upbeat, guaranteed. It's less expensive in the long run to invest a few dollars in the proper container and bring your homemade smoothies with you, rather than relying on the local juice or smoothie bar for your daily fueling.

One note that comes from the experience of some clients. Having all that food packed seems to make you hungrier. It is tempting to eat your lunch by 11:00 a.m. and your mid-afternoon snack before the 3 o'clock hour. You might experiment with doing just that — you may discover that it is a good idea to eat your lunch and snacks at earlier times for optimal mood and performance. But I would suggest that you first drink 8 to 10 ounces of water when you feel ready to dive early into the next snack or meal. Wait fifteen to twenty minutes. If you are still hungry, go for it.

Jennifer Lail, one of the *Post-Intelligencer* participants, participated in a graduate academic program while following the Good Mood Diet. She became legendary for her packed snacks — ribbed for counting out her daily almonds but also revered for eating healthy. Some fellow students actually wondered just what new great snack she was enjoying. "I went to one conference," says Jennifer, laughing, "and I would say about a dozen people commented on my lunches and snacks, asking where did I get the food and where could they buy some!"

Get to know these pit-stop favorites.

Have you ever watched a car go into the pit stop lane at a NASCAR or other car race? The pit crew is working feverishly to refuel, change tires, and do whatever else needs to be done. The idea is be fast and fail-safe. There is no compromising one for the other. Here are some foods to keep in mind for your pit stops. Know where to buy them and you will be ahead of the field.

Jerky: Dried beef, turkey, or salmon serves up a powerful snack for the mid-afternoon blahs or pre-workout fueling. I look for hormone-free varieties of beef and turkey and usually find them at natural groceries. Many of these same stores carry salmon jerky (pick wild over farm-raised) and FishingVessel St.Jude (www.tunatuna.com) carries tuna jerky for variety. Some farmers' markets have jerky booths. Forget the cowboy-food stigma. This is straight-out Good Mood manna.

Chocolate milk: Surprise. I have long told my elite-athlete clients to grab a chocolate milk (usually they like the flavor better than plain) after a workout or game. Now research backs me up. A recent study published in the International Journal of Sport Nutrition and Exercise Metabolism showed that athletes who drank chocolate milk after a workout were able to exercise more intensely during a second workout than those partici-pants who downed a commercial sports drink.[1] The reason is that choco-late milk contains an optimal carb-to-protein ratio to refuel both tired muscles and a taxed brain.

Soy Crisps: Genisoy makes the original snack food product; it comes in various flavors to match up with your hankerings for barbecue, cheese-flavored, ranch dressing, and more. Many natural grocery chains have produced house-brand versions. You will marvel at the snack-food satis-faction of these crisps and yet they stay well within an ideal ratio of bread serving and protein serving for a quick pit stop.

Peanuts in the shell: How cool is this? You can watch a ballgame and stay on the Good Mood plan. Just keep your handful to ten or so peanuts and bring your own apple. I like peanuts in the shell because they take longer to eat and it is easier to savor them.

Apples: An old standby that provides more flavor ranges these days. Don't reach for only the Red Delicious. There are so many great varieties out there: Fuji, Honey Crisp, Braeburn, Granny Smith, Pink Lady, on and on. I like to slice my apples and find some nut butter for dipping. Eating an apple about an hour before your next meal is a great way to control overeating, but I insist that you get some fat and protein with the fruit. Combining is critical to Good Mood maintenance. Add that peanut or almond butter, or the handful of peanuts, or an individual wrapped cheese wedge or stick.

Celery: The Good Mood Diet focuses on feeling great while you lose undesired weight. Good health comes along in the bargain. But I will speak up for the medical power of celery. Many natural health doctors and some high blood pressure researchers tout celery as a protector against hypertension.[2] You can substitute about six celery stalks for your apple.

Edamame: This is the Japanese term for soybeans. I like buying them frozen in the pod (which is discarded like a peanut shell). I boil them for five minutes, then sprinkle on some sea salt, and eat them like popcorn. Kids love them. You can eat them hot or pack them cold for late afternoon. You can find them in most groceries.

Popcorn: Air-popped is the Good Mood version. Don't forget to grab a protein to round out the snack. It is getting easier to find healthy versions (no trans fat and little saturated fat) at convenience stores. Making it at home is still best.

Establish a set of fast-food standards and only compromise to a point.

So this is the deal on fast food. You're always better off packing a sandwich from home. But even in my house that's just not always possible. When I'm making the lifestyle choice to grab a quick sandwich for myself and/ or the kids, I weigh the options: I will not lower my health and mood standards to eat just any fast foods. But sometimes it's worth the stress-reduction to choose from the best options out there. When they're not available, I bring quick food from home, or I stop at the supermarket deli counter and have a sandwich made to order.

As for brand-name burgers, I'm not buying the leaner, healthier McDonald's marketing push, especially with those French fries still dominating the premise. And I certainly am not going to give a thumbs-up to Burger King or Hardees when they have ongoing campaigns for over-the-top burgers. It might be possible to navigate a reasonable baked-potato lunch (with chili) at Wendy's, but you can do better.

Here are three brand-name fast-food choices that fit into our household lifestyle. I am especially untroubled stopping for a Subway meal once or twice per week. In fact, you will note the Good Mood Menus in Chapter 3 include a Subway wrap. What they don't include is the cookie and the soda that go along with the real deal meal. They are no deal, especially when it comes to your mood. Save your money, and your mood, and just get the sandwich and a beverage of either water, milk, or something that is sugar-free.

I have put together this info to help guide you on fast-food choices, including comparable smaller chains or independent stores in your region. This data comes from company websites:

Subway (Favorite Choice)

Choose a six-inch sub (counts as three bread servings) or a wrap (counts as one bread serving) from their extensive menu of items containing 6 grams of fat or less. To increase protein, ask for a double serving of meat, especially if you are regularly working out. Skip the mayonnaise, but do ask for olive oil and load up on the veggies. I pass on the soft drinks and even the baked chips. The chips have less fat, but more carbs, and hardly fewer calories than fried. I'm not a fan of them. I'd rather you had some nuts, veggies, or a piece of fruit. Put baked chips on the special treat list for every once in a while.

Pizza Hut

I picked Pizza Hut because it is everywhere and the nutritional content is reasonable. Some other national chains have more calories and a higher percentage of calories from fat per slice, usually because they load on the cheese. Make it a habit to ask to go easy on the cheese on your pies. Many pizzerias don't seem to understand that adjustment, so I suggest finding one that does for your pizza splurges.

If you go light on the cheese and heavy on the lean protein and vegetable toppings, you are in Good Mood territory. As a family, we order smaller-size pizzas than average but we don't savor it any less. I like filling out a pizza outing with a good homemade soup or green salad at the pizzeria.

Good Mood Choices from Pizza Hut

	Calories	Fat Percent
Medium Chicken Supreme Thin and Crispy (1 slice)	200	30
Medium Veggie Lover's Thin and Crispy (1 slice)	180	33
Medium Cheese Only Hand-Tossed Style (1 slice)	240	29

Medium Ham Hand-Tossed Style (1 slice)	220	23
Medium Chicken Supreme Hand-Tossed Style (1 slice)	230	26
Medium Veggie Lover's Hand-Tossed Style (1 slice)	220	27

Taco Bell

This chain has been rated as a leader in food safety management by industry observers. You can also find a Good Mood lunch or dinner in a pinch. At your own local taquerias, you can do even better — provided you skip the basket of chips (ask for tortillas to dip into salsa and guacamole) and find restaurants that don't use lard in the refried beans and pork carnitas.

Good Mood Choices from Taco Bell

	Calories	Fat Percent
Fresco Style Ranchero Chicken Soft Taco	170	21
Fresco Style Grilled Steak Soft Taco	170	26
Fresco Style Gordita Baja Chicken	230	22
Fresco Style Gordita Baja Steak	230	26
Fresco Style Tostada	200	25
Fresco Style Enchirito Chicken	250	20
Fresco Style Enchirito Steak	250	24
Fresco Style Bean Burrito	370	24
Fresco Style Fiesta Chicken Burrito	340	27
Fresco Style Fiesta Steak Burrito	350	29

Make some adjustments to your restaurant habits.

One of the great features of the Good Mood Diet is by no means do you have to stop dining out. If you study the menus in Chapter 3 or the Feel-Great Foods in Chapter 1, you will quickly determine that many restaurant meals fit into the plan. Not necessarily the portion sizes, but the foods.

On the following page are a few tips on how to eat out and keep the Good Mood momentum.

Don't start on the breadbasket until other food comes to the table. How many times do you realize you filled up too much on bread to enjoy the rest of the meal? Right, too many. Tim Grover, who trained Michael Jordan for all of his championship years in pro basketball and now trains dozens of National Basketball Association stars, tells all of his clients to send the breadbasket back to the kitchen. I say at least wait until other foods (protein and fats) arrive and always dip your bread in olive oil. Plus, decide if you want your bread servings to be actual bread or, say, pasta or mashed potatoes. The more whole grain in the bread, the better.

Share appetizers and order your salad with dressing on the side. At some restaurants, more than half the fun comes from the unusual appetizers offered. Get a taste, but share the dish with your dining companions. Salad dressing on the side is the only way to synchronize your Good Mood; use your fork to mix in the dressing because you will naturally use less. Look for low-fat dressings when possible or the simple but tasty olive oil and balsamic vinegar combination.

Ask for meat and fish sauces on the side. Remember, I am all for Good Mood, so I am not asking you to insult a chef by ordering plain, plain, plain. Figure out how the food is prepared (*deep* and *fry* are not good words together, but *pan-fried* usually passes the Good Mood test) and get the yummy sauces. Just allow yourself to control the sauce portion on your plate.

When ordering pasta, choose the red sauce. White alternatives are typically bringing butter and cream to the experience. In either case, I would regard pasta as a side dish and not the typical main entrée. Whole-grain pasta improves the picture but is rare in most Italian restaurants.

Split desserts for the table. Even sharing among two can save you about 300 calories and, oh, 20 fat grams. Research shows we make room for dessert because we crave a different taste throughout a meal (usually sweet in the matter of dessert). So satisfy your craving without the mood crash that will occur later.

Think combinations. And I don't mean the fried fish-and-shrimp combo. Your plate should have roughly equal parts meat/poultry/fish, steamed veggies, and rice/potato/sweet potato.

Define *splurge* — and then go enjoy yourself.

Vacations are a special case for the Good Mood Diet. I am moved in some ways to urge you to simply let go, and then get back on the Good Mood track when you return to your normal routine. But I hear from so many clients that they enjoyed their vacations and trips more because they stayed on plan.

"The Good Mood Diet works for me, even on vacations," says Louise Goodman, a Good Mood Diet Club member who lost 10 pounds in the first three months, which included an extended trip to Washington, D.C., to visit her eighty-five-year-old mother and other relatives. "When I fall off the plan for a day, I notice I feel lousy."

Nonetheless, you can take mini-vacations from the Good Mood plan and not suffer any lasting consequences. Louise, for instance, says she worries less about the Good Mood parameters when out at an Indian restaurant. Other clients don't make a big deal out of their Good Mood strategies when invited to a dinner party — at least not until everybody asks how it is they are looking so fabulous.

A special case is when visiting family members such as parents or siblings who eat nothing like you do on the Good Mood Diet. Some of my Good Mood Diet Club members wrestle with these issues. My answer is simple. Explain yourself, point out all of the Feel-Great Foods still in your kitchen and, when all else fails, take smaller portions to offset the possible mood drop-off and the inevitable urgings to have second or even third helpings. Even better, buy them a copy of the book and create your own Good Mood Diet Club!

Good Mood Breakthrough Story:

EAT LIKE A CHAMPION, AT HOME OR AWAY

Trish Zuccotti didn't need to lose pounds when we connected in mid-2005. "I wanted to change my body composition," says Trish, who is fifty-nine and a chief accounting officer, senior vice president, and controller at the Expedia travel web site. "I wanted to lose fat."

As an experienced competitive weight lifter — she won the 2005 and 2006 nationals in her age and weight class, then won a Silver Medal at the world championships — Trish knew she might even gain a few pounds of muscle weight. But she also knew changing body composition would provide more power in her arms and legs. The plan surpassed her wildest expectations.

"I was following the same workout routine, which was intense as I got ready for the world championships," says Trish. "I just felt phenomenally stronger on the Good Mood plan. I don't think of it as a diet as much as a new way of eating. My energy level and mental acuity are unbelievably good, especially for my job."

Trish and her coach both give a full measure of credit to the Good Mood Diet for her weight-lifting achievements. "It's the only thing I changed about my routine," Trish says. "I am just so much leaner and stronger. It's just so obvious."

Trish is "fascinated" by how the Good Mood plan has changed her approach to eating. "Instead of eating to lose weight," she says, "I eat to feel good. If I veer off the plan for a couple days, by the third morning I am noticeably more tired. I say, 'OK, time to get in line with the plan,' and two days later I feel fantastic again. It's flabbergasting."

One reason Trish feels so good is she "never goes more than three hours — or four, absolute tops" without eating something. She always carries a stash of nuts and fruits with her. After her highly intense workouts, she is prepared with a recovery snack to eat within thirty minutes of the exercise. Her usual option is plain yogurt and fresh fruit. Sometimes it is cottage cheese with a sliced mango.

She traveled to both Europe and China on business during the past year. She says she always finds a way to make the plan work in other countries. "I bring along some Luna protein bars [which are not too heavy on the carbs], plus dried fruit and my usual nuts. But the first day in a new place I look for the local equivalent of a deli or small grocery to pick up fresh fruit and other Good Mood snacks."

Trish changed jobs in 2005 after twenty-two years and a high comfort level with another employer. "I don't think I could have handled the new job and pace very well without [the Good Mood plan]," she says.

There's yet one more bonus for Trish at home. Her sixty-year-old hus-band, Andrew, had "never been one to work out." But watching his wife break through with the Good Mood plan inspired him. He started follow-ing the Good Mood template in January 2006 and lost twenty pounds in the first three months. "He told me one day 'I just haven't had this much energy in my whole life,' " says Trish. "Andrew is somebody who would never have believed it if he didn't experience it himself."

6

GOOD MOOD X-FACTORS: EXERCISE AND REST

I am a big fan of the truth. A huge fan. The truth is there is no diet plan that will help you lose weight, make you feel great, and keep the weight off for a lifetime without including some exercise.

In fact, I work only one-on-one with clients who work out regularly because I know that diet alone won't do it for you. If someone calls me and doesn't want to include exercise in his/her plan, then I refer them to someone else. I want every client that I work with to have a success story.

Regular exercise is going to get you the results you dream about — and keep that dream a reality. Diet and exercise are both essential parts of the Good Mood equation.

Same goes for sleep and rest, the other Good Mood X-Factor. You don't lose weight while you sleep, but you can't lose weight if you don't get enough sleep. Sleep deprivation translates to higher amounts of stress hormones, especially cortisol, in your blood levels day and night. More cortisol means less fat burning. So staying up late, whether to be productive or unwind from the day, could be sabotaging your weight-loss goals. That's because one of cortisol's "duties" in the body is to prevent you from burning fat, to ensure survival during lean times. The body mechanism was more useful in primitive times, but remains operative nonetheless. The truth is adequate sleep is necessary for weight loss.

One more thing: Getting enough rest for Good Mood includes taking some "down time" during the day. There is ample psychology research to show taking short breaks from work or tasks every forty minutes will renew mental efficiency and training.[1] You need to rest the brain just like you might give your arms and shoulders a spell while chopping wood or lifting weights.

Ergonomic experts urge computer users to stand and stretch every twenty minutes. The concept is to avoid repetitive stress injuries (especially to the wrists) and relieve the spine and neck. Plus, you take better care of your eyes that way. It's all about recharging the Good Mood energy cell.

The first Good Mood X-Factor is the hidden exercise in our days.

Let's start with a couple of stories about how exercise can be part of every day, whether you make it to the gym or not. Trish Zuccotti is a champion competitive weight lifter who doesn't need my advice to determine a workout program. But we have collaborated on improving her energy levels through nutrition (you can read about it in a Good Mood Breakthrough Story, page 127).

Trish called one day a few weeks before a major competition. She was having trouble making weight in her class, meaning she was a few pounds heavier than allowed. She was perplexed because weight control had never been an issue.

We determined her Good Mood Diet choices had been consistent over the last year. So what's different, I asked her. Not the food, not the workouts, seemingly nothing.

"Tell me about your new job," I said. "Do you walk much around the office?"

Her answer was, well, not really at all. It turns out everything is on one floor, compared to Trish's former office, where she went up and down stairs much more frequently. Plus, Trish is a vice president these days, meaning she goes on fewer client calls and people come more often to see her.

"That's the difference," I said. "You need to walk up and down the stairs at your office four times a day."

Trish did just that and her weight started coming down.

I told Trish I knew the feeling. When our family moved from Cleveland to Seattle, our new house was a one-level. Instead of working in a basement office and running up to the second floor to go to the bathroom, now I didn't have to go far. Nothing else changed in my diet or exercise routine. Within four to six months, I had gained 5 pounds.

Set a goal of 10,000 steps per day.

The lesson is there is exercise in your day of which you might not even be aware. Setting a goal of taking 10,000 steps per day can increase your exercise awareness and decrease any tendency to gain weight.

Some of my clients find the 10,000 steps to be no problem because they walk as part of a commute, live in highly walkable neighborhoods, or maybe walk their dogs two or three times per day. Other clients and Good Mood Diet Club members find the 10,000 mark to be almost impossible. I urge them to keep looking for more steps in their daily routines — and they always find a way to reach 10,000.

The 10,000-step mark has been studied by exercise scientists, who say that someone who takes this many lefts and rights each day is an active person "exercising" enough to lose weight or maintain weight loss. No matter if those steps are simply part of your normal day's route or specifically added as a brisk walk or recreational hike.

For example, a University of Tennessee study found middle-aged women who took at least 10,000 steps per day were much more likely to have healthy body weight and body fat percentages. Women who took 6,000 or less steps had an average of 44 percent body fat and generally fell well into the overweight category[2].

Moreover, in a 2005 study, researchers with the American College of

Sports Medicine worked with fifty-eight physically inactive women, giving them a choice of setting a 10,000-step goal or taking a thirty-minute walk each day. The women choosing the steps goal averaged 11,775 on days when they met their goals, compared to 9,505 steps for the thirty-minute walkers. Perhaps as importantly, on days when the women didn't meet their goals, the 10,000-step group still significantly outperformed the thirty-minute walk group by more than 2,000 steps (7,780 steps to 5,597 steps).

The typical American takes about 6,000 steps per day in their lives, which leaves about 4,000 steps for a brisk thirty-minute walk[3]. One problem, most people don't find the time or inclination to take that walk. The highly beneficial 4,000 steps — or roughly two miles — vanish while that last five pounds in generally healthy people stays put.

Invest in a pedometer.

No doubt too many people have stationary bikes with clothes hanging on them, or yoga gear that is stored in back of the closet. But I would like to be so bold as to urge you to spend a bit of money on a good pedometer. My favorite brand is New Lifestyles (www.new-lifestyles.com), which offers a range of pedometers from twenty-five dollars and up. My favorite models are in their NL series, and the NL-2000 has been shown in published research studies to be a reliable pedometer for all body types. I have tried some of the cheaper models from other brands and found them to be uneven in counting steps. One note: More employers and insurance carriers are running special programs to promote pedometers; ask around at your office.

The New Lifestyles pedometers can be linked to your computer for easy log entries. But my primary goal in persuading you to buy a pedometer is acquainting yourself with just how much hidden exercise is in your day — or is possible in your day. You can use it to determine just how many steps you cover in such activities as walking your kids to school, shopping at the grocery store, or working on the lawn and garden.

Take the stairs every chance you get.

Kelly Brownell, a health researcher at Yale who specializes in obesity, once conducted an experiment that showed he could triple the number of users (albeit still low) on one stairwell by posting this sign at the ground floor: "Your heart needs the exercise, here's your chance!"

Taking the stairs is an efficient calorie-burning activity, on par with trail hiking or a vigorous weight-training workout. Some personal trainers say their clients can lose five to ten pounds in a year simply by taking the stairs when sensible — nobody is suggesting you climb, say, twenty-four stories to reach your office even if that would be an excellent workout. From my viewpoint, using stairs rather than elevators or escalators is a must for fast-tracking Good Mood.

Don't forget good technique on those stairs. Tim Burnham, assistant professor of exercise science at Central Washington University, recommends not using the railings ("except to maintain balance") when taking the stairs. Holding onto the railing lowers the heart rate and burns fewer calories.

A 2005 American Heart Association conference highlighted some intriguing results of hill workouts, which certainly can be accomplished on stairs if your usual walking or running route is flat. Austrian researchers studied a group of hikers in the Alps and found that uphill hiking clears fats (especially triglycerides) from the blood quicker, while downhill hiking reduces blood sugar more effectively (an argument for taking the stairs down too). Hiking either way lowered cholesterol of the participants.

See you at the stairwell.

Add intensity to your exercise regimen.

Here's a breakthrough moment for people who are in great shape. They have figured out that the most effective workouts incorporate bouts of intensity. Runners who perform speed workouts or "intervals" discover that race events come easier. Weight lifters who push (safely) to the point of exhaustion realize the best results in muscle toning and weight control. Every form of exercise has room for heightened intensity.

Consider the rule of thumb that the proper exercise intensity is somewhere between easy conversation with a training partner (who might be
on foot or riding a bike) and breathing so hard you can't utter a word. I
advise that you be able to converse but not without some laboring. Trust
me, if you add intensity to even one workout each week — or 2,000 steps
per day for the 10,000-step goal — you will notice a pleasant boost in
mood and accelerate your weight loss along with it.

Of course, one way to intensify your exercise routine is develop a regular habit. The Institute of Medicine recommends an hour of daily exercise.

OK, you can stop snickering now. That's why I have talked here about
counting steps of the day with a pedometer. If you can find the time for
additional activities, some of the recommendations include brisk walking, running, cycling, swimming, using a piece of cardiovascular exercise
equipment, or dancing. If pickup basketball or social league volleyball
might be your thing, go for it.

The American College of Sports Medicine suggests that cardiovascular training is only part of total fitness. You also need strength training
(usually with weights) and flexibility exercises. For the best results in the
Good Mood Diet, I endorse two or three cardio workouts and two or
three weight-training workouts each week, along with getting 10,000
steps every day. An equally positive Good Mood strategy is stretching for
at least five to ten minutes every other day. You might be able to combine
some of these workouts to save time, such as using a Pilates class for a
strength-stretching combination or trying a Body Pump class that twins
cardio and strength work.

Whatever your exercise choice, be sure to follow the right techniques.

There's an axiom among exercise scientists about what is the "best" physical activity: "The best exercise is the one you do."

The Good Mood Diet allows plenty of choices in what motivates you
to be physically active — and doesn't require a gym membership or
hours of drudgery. But I do urge you to follow proper form in whatever

you do, even if it is walking. Find a knowledgeable friend, seek out a coach or trainer, take a class. Because learning proper technique prepares you for more intense workouts, which ultimately represent the great fitness "secret" shared by trainers and elite athletes alike.

Tim Grover, who trained Michael Jordan during the championship years and now supervises workouts for dozens of pro basketball stars, has always used this slogan: "Even the best athletes can get better." He achieves that by turning up the intensity of his clients' exercise programs.

While public health officials contend any exercise is better than being sedentary, the deep-root message is we have to push our bodies and mindsets to get in the best condition. It is wise to start slow — and seek a physician's approval if you have any health concerns — but eventually you want to be feeling the intensity. It will pay off with lasting weight loss and higher energy. But be patient with yourself.

"The first step is to be consistent," says Gregory Florez, founder of Fit Advisor.com, an online personal training and coaching company based in Salt Lake City. "Make time for your activity. Then do it correctly from the first step or lift to the last."

Florez recommends that his clients add strength training to their workout weeks, even if they are dedicated runners, cyclists, or walkers. It leads to more results, especially if your primary goal is weight loss or endurance. Exhaustion, which doesn't sound fun but is rewarding in a good fatigue sort of way, is the objective.

"That means you complete every repetition with good form," says Florez, "but have no gas left in the tank when you are done."

There is an unsung benefit in your focus on good form and on working the muscles to full load. You forget any troubles or problems for those present moments, even if it is for a few seconds. The stress can fall away like the perspiration in your shirt. You are free. Exercise becomes a Good Mood X-Factor.

Make the connection between mood and exercise.

This book is all about connecting food and mood. Exercise is another strong and valuable influence on mood. Think of it as like another positive role model in a teenager's life, whether that person is a coach, teacher, or even a peer. Parents with teens know they need all the help and support they can get. Same goes for staying in Good Mood territory.

A formidable body of research has connected mood and exercise. What's exciting is the evidence is increasingly based on the objective measurements and observations available through functional brain imaging techniques. Researchers can literally see the "happy" parts of the brain light up on their screens. This imaging technique joins the long-accepted standardized self-surveys to gauge mood.

Gregory Berns, a researcher who teaches psychiatry and behavioral science at Emory University in Atlanta, has been going one step further. He believes that the striatum, a small bit of tissue in the lower brain, is the cornerstone of being satisfied in life. Using cutting-edge scanning technology, Berns has studied the interaction of dopamine, the hormone the brain produces when anticipating pleasure, and cortisol, which as we have discussed in previous chapters is the stress hormone. His conclusion is the chemical bath of the striatum leads each of us to seek out satisfaction in novel physical ways, whether it is walking on nature trails, becoming a master gardener, or hitting the perfect golf shot.

Physical activity boosts the serotonin levels in our brain, leading to brighter moods and clearer thinking. Being active also rings up mood-altering chemicals called endorphins, which are the body's natural opiates. You may have heard endorphins associated with a "runner's high."

Although some research indicates that endorphins are only elevated with peak levels of exercise, there is no question that exercise increases your overall energy levels and can promote an overall sense of well-being that overflows from the gym or walking path into your home and professional lives.

Here's a 2006 study that was published in the official journal of the American College of Sports Medicine[4]. Researchers at the University of

Texas showed that even a single bout of exercise — thirty minutes of walking on a treadmill — can improve the mood of volunteer patients suffering from clinical depression. The participants were not regular exercisers and were not taking antidepressants for their conditions.

The control group engaged in "quiet rest" that included leaving home and interacting with others. Both groups of participants reported lower negative feelings such as tension, anger, and fatigue. But only the one-bout exercise group reported higher scores for vigor and well-being. The Texas researchers reasoned that "many people with depression attempt to self-medicate with alcohol, caffeine, or tobacco to manage their daily routine. Low- to moderate-intensity exercise appears to be an alternate way to manage depression — one that doesn't come with such negative health consequences."

This study breaks new ground because it shows an immediate mood boost. Previous studies have only tracked long-term lifts in mood. Expect this field of study to virtually explode in the next decade.

The second Good Mood X-Factor is the necessity of proper rest for losing pounds and keeping them off.

Getting enough rest is the weak link of the fitness triumvirate, far less considered than physical activity or eating healthfully — but no less important. There are two facets to this Good Mood X-Factor. One is sleep. You know that one: bed, pillows, darkened room, get seven to eight hours.

The other facet is rest as defined as time away from the health club or walking trail to allow for proper muscle recovery. Researchers believe muscles that are worked strenuously to exhaustion (weight-lifting sets, intensive sprint workouts) need thirty-six to forty-eight hours to recover and rebuild.

The benefits of getting enough sleep is not news. My contribution to the discussion is to inform you that cheating yourself out of sleep can also block your ability to lose weight. We have talked early in this chapter about how the body goes into a survival mode when we don't get enough sleep. The exact amount of "enough" is debatable and personal, but it is my view from the research literature that seven to eight hours is the proper amount, even when we get older and think we need a bit less sleep time.

That same sleep research offers up some valuable tips about healthful sleep hygiene. Some highlights:

- Try to go to bed and wake up at the same time, even on weekends. People with a set bedtime/wake-up schedule seem to function best — and adjust easier when overnight has to be shorter because of travel, work, family duties, etc.
- The most important sleep habit is waking up at the same time. It resets the bio-chronological clocks in our bodies.
- Be sure your room is completely dark, at least to allow the seven to eight hours of sleep. This allows the brain to produce the ideal amounts of serotonin and melatonin, the latter a sleep hormone that encourages restful sleep and downtime for the brain.
- Keep the room a bit cool. This will cut down on waking up because you are overheated.
- Be careful about drinking alcohol too close to bedtime. Research shows alcohol makes us drowsy for bedtime but disturbs the second half of the night's rest, when the most REM (rapid-eye movement) deep-sleep minutes are logged.
- Avoid any form of exercise at least two hours before bed. Working out increases body temperature, which makes it harder to fall asleep.

I will add one to the list. Drink your Good Mood cup of hot cocoa before bed. It contains tryptophan, which is an amino acid that at night-time leads the body to feel appropriately drowsy and relaxed.

Patrick D'Amelio, one of the *Seattle Post-Intelligencer* diet group members, realized quickly how the Good Mood eating plan and the suggested 10,000 steps (he did some of his on exercise machines) were positively impacting his rest pattern. "I slept better right away," recalls Patrick. "I started getting up an hour or two before the alarm clock rang and feeling great."

Eat and drink for muscle recovery.

One of the biggest trends in sports nutrition is eating for muscle recovery. It means replenishing your body after exercise to maximize muscle growth and fat loss. You might think it is contradictory to eat right after working out, but that is exactly the time for the boost we all desire in mood and fat burning.

You may have read or heard that muscles need mega-protein after workouts to build the most muscle. Not true, but protein plus carbohydrates is critically important after exercise. As little as 20 grams of high quality protein (more is not better) will accelerate protein synthesis in the muscles following exercise. Although protein powders and amino-acid supplements are not absolutely essential, liquid forms of nutrition get to the muscle more quickly after exercise compared to solid foods. That's why I recommend a smoothie with whey protein after a morning workout (when it's possible to exercise that time of day) in the menu plan every day. The whey protein feeds your muscles and lifts your mood at the same time. And the milk contains a natural mixture of protein and carbohydrates that gets you ready to work out again tomorrow.

Here is the regimen I give to all my clients and suggest for anyone starting a regular workout program:

Fluids: Drink at least 8 ounces of water in the hour before exercise, then consume 7 to 10 ounces for every twenty minutes of activity. If your exercise session lasts more than an hour, sip on sports drinks instead of water. After the workout, replace each pound lost (this is about the only time I recommend getting on a scale) with 16 to 20 ounces of water or sports drink.

Meals: Eat a meal (breakfast or lunch) at least four hours before exercise. This is best-picture for providing carbohydrates for the muscles. If you are a first-thing-in-the-morning exerciser, experiment with a light snack of a glass of fat-free milk, a low-sugar yogurt, or a slice of bread with an ounce of cheese to fuel your body without taxing your digestive tract. And don't forget the fluids.

If your workout is later in the day, be sure to get the same sort of slow-release combination snack thirty to ninety minutes before exertion. A cup of yogurt is an effective pre-workout snack. You can eat it as close as thirty minutes before exercise time, provided your digestive system can handle it.

In any case, after your exercise make it your business to get fast-release carbohydrates: sports drinks work great or foods high on the glycemic index, such as a plain bagel, banana, or pretzels within a half-hour and then again two hours later. You also *must* get some protein at this time to maximize the results of exercise. This is when the muscle growth and fat loss happens. Ideally your snack will be in liquid form, because it will get to your muscles faster. That's why I've included the smoothie as your post-workout snack. You can take one of your fruits from later in the day and mix it in, too. I recommend about 20 grams of protein and at least 12 grams of carbs (it can go much higher the more fit you are and the longer your workout). If you eat a bagel, add some turkey and a glass of milk to it. The post–two hour carbs can be part of a meal such as pasta with turkey meatballs.

Memo to your sweet tooth: Immediately after exercise is the best time to partake in some or all of the added 6 teaspoons of sugar during each week of the Feel Great While You Lose Weight phase outlined in Chapter 3.

Don't forget your cool-down.

When you add intensity to your workouts, it is important to allow time for cooldown period lasting ten to twenty minutes. Continuing light exercise for five to ten minutes after your strenuous walk helps the body remove the lactic acid in muscles that leads to soreness and stiffness.

Follow up the light exercise with five to ten minutes of stretching. Many researchers and trainers now contend we get the most gains in flexibility and injury prevention by stretching after the muscles are warm[5]. Just remember to maintain proper techniques.

Good Mood Breakthrough Story:

BECOMING A MORNING EATER

With two young kids at home and nearing fifty years of age, Sharon Lee Hamilton is looking for all of the energy she can muster. Her commitment to Good Mood breakfasts makes a vibrant difference in her life — and represents a healthy ritual each day.

"I basically have three breakfasts that I eat," says Sharon. "One of the fastest is that I boil and peel eggs the night before and refrigerate. In the morning I microwave the egg and have half an English muffin. I use olive oil for fat on the egg, and have either half a grapefruit or orange, and yogurt. (I precook enough eggs for my children to eat also.)"

Another option for Sharon is to put frozen fruit in the blender, generally blueberries, with soy milk (protein) and yogurt (milk). She blends and adds flax meal, then toasts half an English muffin.

"I guess I like English muffins more than I realized because the third breakfast I eat a lot is that I combine ricotta cheese with fruit juice–sweetened cherry jam and the flax meal," says Sharon. "I eat the mixture spread on an English muffin with fat-free milk."

Sharon admits to feeling more challenged for lunch and dinner, but Good Mood snacks are easy to fit into her day with two youngsters. She sees the positives in carrying out some if not all Good Mood strategies. "I lost four pounds early on the diet, then gained it back," says Sharon. "But here's the important thing. I haven't gained weight since adopting our second child. I know I would have put on some pounds without the Good Mood Diet."

7

GOOD MOOD MOMENTUM: KEEPING IT GOING

I don't know about you, but I need some "me" time in my day or week. So I turn off my cell phone during exercise time. I know my kids are in a safe place (with trusted adults, in school, at camp, etc.) and I determine to let go of my other life responsibilities for the next hour.

The break renews my spirit and lets me concentrate on the workout. I get a double boost in mood.

As my clients tell me over and over, their energy levels soar in the first weeks of the Good Mood Diet. The wonderful fact is that you can keep that Good Mood momentum going for a lifetime. You won't feel deprived or ever hungry. You will connect your food with how you feel, which is a much more powerful motivator than what the scale reads.

And here's one of the best parts. When you veer off the plan for whatever reason, the Good Mood Diet will be right there to support you. Even the day of the splurge or during a week when life's deadlines pull at you, the Good Mood strategy focuses on making sure you get your Feel-Great Foods and not dwelling on any "slips." For instance, I want you to end your day with a hot cocoa, no matter what. How great is that?

Plus, when you get back to the highly livable Good Mood plan you will feel better and more energetic within one day. After two days, you will feel supercharged and understand that Good Mood Momentum is at your beckoning.

Now that you have all of this Good Mood energy, I say let your creative self out to play. You can use the energy to work on the important things in your life, whether it might be relationships, staking a career move, or digging into a home project. Use that Good Mood energy to your highest advantage. Here are some Good Mood Momentum builders:

Forget your bathroom scale; your clothes will tell you.

When Paula Burke, a mother of two toddlers, was participating in the Good Mood Diet as part of the *Seattle Post-Intelligencer* group, she didn't even get on a scale from early January until Easter. That's when she stepped on one in her mother's guest bathroom. Bam, she lost ten pounds, something she guessed because her clothing size was down a size or two and she was fitting into her "skinny jeans" again.

You don't have to throw out your bathroom scale, unless you find it too irresistible to step on every day. One way to establish and keep momentum going is to find another way to mark your progress. Our weight can naturally fluctuate a few pounds during a day or week. What's more, if you begin an exercise program, particularly training with weights, you might actually gain a few pounds but lose inches around your waist and hips.

Get to know your taste buds.

We all know the advertising slogan, "There's always room for Jell-O." Just how is it that no matter how full we might be, we can always eat dessert if it's put in front of us?

It's because our brains crave variety and dessert provides a sweet, intense flavor that might not otherwise be part of the meal[1]. The Good

Mood meals and snacks typically include a serving of fruit, such as a sectioned orange at dinner or ¼ cup of dried cherries for a mid-afternoon pick-me-up. Chapter 8 provides dozens of recipes, including an ample supply of healthy sweets and desserts. You can indulge your sweet tooth and those variety-seeking taste buds — but without later crashing from a sugar high.

There's always room for variety. When you are out with friends, you don't have to spoil a moment of fun by skipping dessert. Just ask for one dessert and three or four forks. What your brain craves is just a few bites, not the whole thing. Try it, you will see.

Consider yourself an eater, not a dieter.

When you come home at eight o'clock at night and you're hungry, I don't want you thinking about what you can't eat. I want you happy to focus on what you still *need* to eat to feed your mood and brain — both that evening and the next morning.

To that end, no food is entirely off-limits. Always combine starches or what I call bread servings with protein and healthy fat. When you eat crackers, enjoy them, savor them, but with some peanut butter. Add a cheese stick to your apple snack. There's nothing wrong with a hamburger when you get home at eight, just put it on a whole-wheat bun.

Other foods that fit into the Good Mood Diet: Steak, dark-meat turkey, corn bread, chili, Asian stir-fry, oatmeal, lox, cream cheese, whole-wheat English muffin, barbecued pork, mango, green tea, Soy Crisps, a glass of milk, your favorite whole-grain cold cereal, tacos, Japanese udon soup, an omelet, corn on the cob, red wine and — yes! — dark chocolate.

In fact, I want you to end your day with a delicious cup of genuine hot cocoa. Don't skip it, thinking you are being "extra healthy or good." Quite the contrary. You are messing with the Good Mood Template. The cocoa helps you get a good night's sleep, feel decadent, and wake up with energy. Some Good Mood eaters make it a nighttime ritual with a spouse or partner. I say make it mandatory, even on nights when you, ahem, may have overindulged.

Forget all negative research about eggs.

I urge you to eat one egg a day, including the yolk. The only exceptions are individuals under strict orders from a physician to eliminate eggs or anyone with an egg allergy.

If you want an omelet or larger egg dish, add egg whites to the first whole egg. The yolk might have some fat but it's where all the brain nutrients — and I mean supernutrients — are stored. Just this egg-a-day habit can change your mornings and entire days.

One of my Good Mood Diet Club members fretted a bit about her newfound egg-a-day habit because she was going on a trip home to see her mother. I bypassed the opportunity to point out the club member was a fifty-plus adult who could make her own eating decisions, thank you, and instead suggested just explaining to Mom that the Good Mood plan has a low and healthy amount of cholesterol in its daily menu options, even with the egg [2].

You might get a similar frown when you snack on nuts or munch on some peanuts (technically legumes) during a ballgame. Tell Mom it is healthy to eat nuts or nut butter every day. Peanuts are just the start. Stretch out to almonds, walnuts, hazelnuts, cashews. Nuts are not a negative. I say you *need* to eat them!

Try keeping a log, at least when you need it.

Research shows many dieters claim the most important thing they did for success was to write down what they ate and how they exercised every day [3]. You can check out Appendix B to see a sample Good Mood Log. When people keep records of what they eat every day, they eat more healthfully, lose weight, and find more success at keeping the weight off. And if they happen to gain a few pounds, they go right back to recording their food and exercise habits to easily lose the extra weight.

Along with recording what you have done, I want you to record how you feel. That's really the bottom line of the Good Mood Diet. If you can look back on your days and see that you felt best on the days that you followed the plan, then you will be motivated to stick with it. The best way to change old habits into new ones with healthy momentum is to keep track of what you do. It's your personal "look out" system, as in "look out, I'm dragging or feeling down."

Confession time: I don't keep a daily log. It's not my style, never has been. But I do temporarily keep a Good Mood Log in two instances.

The first instance is to make sure I'm on track when I anticipate a stressful period ahead. My tendency is to not eat when I am stressed, versus eat too much. As we have discussed throughout this book, not eating during the day yields adverse results for mood and any weight-control goals. Keeping a log during times of high stress — it only takes minutes to log my food and exercise during a day — gets me to pay attention to what I eat and how I react so I don't grab for junk or skip eating all together.

Other times I am less diligent about my diet. Now I admit my "deep end" is still shallow by many standards, but it is still my relative deviation. When I do go off the deep end and start not feeling so good, that's the other time I keep a log for a day or three. I use the log to get back on track and in the Good Mood mindset.

Vow to be "dynamically consistent."

Indiana University psychology professor Jerome Busemeyer has his own take on why people decide, say, at bedtime, to work out the next morning, then roll over when the alarm clock buzzes. Or why they decide not to maintain the momentum of feeling good.

"Most of us are dynamically inconsistent," says Busemeyer, taking a late-day break at his Decision Research Laboratory on IU's campus in Bloomington. "The person who made the decision at night is not the same person who is making the decision in the morning."

Outside of brushing our teeth or reading some pages of a book, it doesn't seem that we can change that much over night. Busemeyer explains that "planning decisions" such as the nighttime vow to exercise the next morning, are less controlled by emotional consequences (feeling tired, pain, not wanting to face the day quite yet) and more linked to benefits (more energy, sense of accomplishment, stress reduction). But when we face a "final decision" there is a tangle of emotions that can grip us.

University of Washington radiologist Dr. Dean Shibata authored a 2001 study that aligns with Busemeyer's research. Shibata found that emotional and rational parts of the brain are closely related, more than previously believed by neuroscientists. Radiology imaging technology allows for researchers like Shibata to see brain activity on a screen when asking volunteer subjects to make decisions.

"Our research supports the idea that every time you have to make choices in your personal life, you need to 'feel' the projected emotional outcome of each choice," says Shibata.

The Good Mood Diet and its momentum affords the chance to become "consistently dynamic." You don't eat to lose weight, you eat to feel good. You connect the emotional and rational parts of the brain. It all adds up to Good Mood Momentum.

Good Mood Breakthrough Story

WHISTLE WHILE YOU EAT FOR GOOD MOOD

During her early weeks on the Good Mood Diet, Paula Burke admits to "whistling a lot" more. Even work projects with "challenging deadlines" didn't stress her out or stop the happy tunes.

Paula was part of the *Seattle Post-Intelligencer* group. She and fellow group member Jennifer Lail became fast friends and often traded notes and experiences. They formed their own sort of Good Mood Diet Club, an idea that I have used to start other groups around the country. You can find out more at www.goodmooddiet.com.

Here's a "listen-in" on a conversation among Paula, Jennifer, and my coauthor, Bob:

BOB: Can you two talk about what surprised you the most on this plan?

JENNIFER: I have been delighted and surprised by the increase in energy I experienced within five days of starting the plan, and that something as [seemingly] simple as nutritional balance has yielded what seems to be a complete cure for my depression.

I used to feel absolutely starved and grumpy by the time I got on the evening ferry, but now feel that I can happily wait to have dinner when I get home. My sleep has improved, which I attribute to reducing my alcohol intake.

PAULA: Vegetables can be the hardest thing to get when you are traveling!

I had to remind myself what Susan said from the start: Even if you eat something that isn't "on the plan," you still need all the stuff on the plan. So just because I had a piece of banana bread at a friend's house, I still needed to have the whole-grain servings for the day too. That took a little while to accept.

BOB: Talk about the supermarket tour you took with Susan.

JENNIFER: The supermarket tour was a real eye-opener in terms of realizing how much sugar is added to foods I previously thought of as healthy. I was surprised to learn from Susan that the average American consumes 20 teaspoons of sugar a day, and some may eat up to 50.

BOB: What habits will stick with you the most?

PAULA: I realized that some of my eating habits were related to stress. I have tried to remind myself that eating in the car or at my desk doesn't give me a chance to enjoy my food. If I am going to have some chocolate, I don't want it to be an absent-minded experience.

JENNIFER: The elimination of sugar has had the most impact on me. On the few days where I deviated from this part of the plan, my whole body felt terrible.

As my energy increased, so did the frequency and length of my sessions at the gym. I always carry an apple, V8 Juice, dried fruit, and nuts with me in case I get stuck on a late ferry, and precooked prawns are my new fast food at the grocery if I am in a pinch.

I am no longer attracted to anything made with white flour. I have substituted all-natural Stevia for sugar, and now drink decaffeinated green tea instead of coffee (and I carry a supply of tea bags with me).

BOB: Did you meet goals for yourself? Surpass them?

JENNIFER: My goal was to stick closely to the food combinations and timing suggested by Susan in hopes of increasing my energy level and combating depression. Both happened. I cannot imagine going back to my old ways — there is great freedom in feeling positive about your physical body and emotional health.

PAULA: I wanted to incorporate more exercise, cushion myself from the winter blahs, and stabilize the weight that was creeping back up. I think my goals shifted slightly. I definitely kept my weight in check but that really seems secondary to the way I feel following the Good Mood plan. I am much more aware of how active I am now. I am fitting in as much activity as I can with a young child at home. I am walking to my office occasionally, jumping rope on the patio for twenty minutes, or walking my older child to school. I found that even a short walk in the course of my day will bump me up to 10,000 steps on my pedometer.

BOB: What was the hardest part, what might block you from maintaining Good Mood Momentum?

PAULA: I never *loved* the smoothie. I ended up doing milk and turkey jerky a lot of the time. I will do the smoothie if I am at home but it's not my favorite.

I would say I followed the plan pretty well in terms of eating the portions for a day but that I probably doubled the sugar allotment for the week most weeks after the first month on the plan (alcohol was the culprit). Nonetheless, I think I definitely made different choices than previously. I was much more aware of checking in with myself, "Do I really want some wine?"

JENNIFER: I spent nine days at a backcountry medicine class, and
was not able to follow the timing exactly for each meal.
Despite getting plenty of exercise during those days and
following the plan as much as possible, I could feel a big
difference in overall well-being, and was glad to get back to
my Good Mood routine and timing.

Sticking to two glasses of red wine a week was tricky at
times — it made me very aware of the prominent role of
alcohol in social settings and how much I used to rely on a
nightly glass of wine to relax. Now that personal
decompression comes from daily cardio workouts and hot
cocoa before bed.

8

GOOD MOOD RECIPES:
FROM SOUP TO SMOOTHIES

Pull up a chair and dig into these Good Mood recipes. This eating plan is about feeling great, which means having fun with friends and loved ones who want to share a meal with you. This chapter is full of good ideas about sharing the fun — and the Good Mood.

What's more, you will find fuel in these recipes, whether it is a different idea for breakfast or deciding to make a treat to satisfy your Good Mood sweet tooth.

The most important thing to remember about these recipes is that they are strictly a starting point. You can adjust your own recipes for the Good Mood boost or mix and match your favorites from this list. The idea is to give you a launch point for improving mood, not to pin you down.

On the other hand, I remember years ago attending a nutrition conference and hearing Dr. William Castelli, lead researcher of the famed Framingham heart studies, talk about food habits of the American family. He estimated that the typical family uses about ten recipes over and over. I think you'll find a number of recipes in this chapter that you can put into your Good Mood rotation.

You will notice there is a Good Mood analysis after each recipe. This feature guides you through the dishes with your daily template of food group servings in mind, as explained in Chapter 3. In many cases, the analysis also includes a count of dietary fiber, which helps you feel less hungry and works to promote health.

There are no breakout salmon recipes in this chapter, mostly because I cook it so often that I don't think of my preparations as recipes, but only a part of normal life. Here are two very easy recipes for salmon that I use regularly. I do on occasion get fancy with my salmon, but this pair of preparations goes a long way in my house:

1. Place salmon in microwave-safe dish (I like to use a steak here, rather than a fillet). Drizzle with olive oil and sprinkle with dill and a little good-tasting salt and lemon juice. Cover and microwave on high for 3 to 4 minutes, depending on the weight and thickness of the piece. Remove and let sit for a minute or two; serve with a lemon wedge. This is so great because it doesn't smell up your house, and it's so easy to prepare a serving just for one.

2. On the grill or in the broiler: I like to use a fillet here, rather than a steak. Rub kosher salt into the skin. Turn over and spread a little olive oil into the flesh, salt very slightly. Place on grill or under the broiler and cook for 7 to 12 minutes, depending on the weight and thickness of the piece. It should begin to get crispy around the edges of the skin. Remove and serve with a lemon wedge. Of all the fancy ways to make salmon, this is still my favorite, and it's *so* easy.

Enjoy the recipes — and don't hesitate to send us your own Good Mood variations and favorites at www.goodmooddiet.com.

Black Bean Salsa Soup

This soup is an easy and delicious way to get beans in your diet. You can adjust the heat by using mild or spicy salsa. And check out the fiber content!

   1 large can (29 ounces) low-sodium black beans, rinsed
   1 jar (16 ounces) medium-heat salsa
   1 can (10 ounces) low-sodium chicken broth
   Optional garnishes: sliced jalapeno, chopped olives,
       chopped avocado, low-fat sour cream

In a blender, puree half the beans with the salsa and broth. Add the remaining beans, transfer to a saucepan, and bring to a boil. Simmer 5 minutes. Garnish and serve.

Makes 4 servings.

Good Mood analysis

Each serving contains 1 bread; 1 vegetable; 1 very lean protein; 10 grams dietary fiber.

Potato Leek Soup

This soup is a delicious way to get in your alliums (vegetables from the onion family) and still keep you kissable. This is a very thick soup. It remains hot for a long time, so don't burn your tongue. If you want a white soup, use only the white of the leeks.

8 large potatoes, diced
4 leeks, cleaned and sliced
2 tablespoons olive oil
8 cups vegetable broth
1 can (12 ounces) evaporated skim milk
salt and white pepper to taste
minced chives

Sauté the potatoes and leeks in olive oil until the leeks are tender. Add the broth and bring to a boil. Cover and simmer on low until the potatoes are tender. Stir in the evaporated milk and heat through. Season with salt and pepper.

Whip the soup with a submergible electric wand or place in a blender and blend to the desired consistency. Serve topped with minced chives.

Makes 16 servings.

Good Mood analysis

Each serving contains 2 breads; 2 vegetables; 4 grams dietary fiber.

Manhattan Clam Chowder

Savor the benefits of both vegetable soup and clam chowder — but with little fat.

2 onions, diced

4 stalks celery, diced

2 leeks, cleaned and diced

2 tablespoons olive oil

1 large can (28 ounces) chopped tomatoes in juice

1 can (10.5 ounces) tomato puree

1 pound potatoes, peeled and cubed

1 teaspoon dried thyme

1½ quarts clam juice

1 can (20 ounces) clams

2 teaspoons Worcestershire sauce

1 to 2 teaspoons Tabasco

Salt and pepper, to taste

In a stock pot, sauté the onions, celery, and leeks in the oil until tender. Add the tomatoes, tomato puree, potatoes, thyme, and clam juice. Cook 30 minutes, or until the potatoes are tender.

Add the clams, Worcestershire sauce, and Tabasco. Season with salt and pepper. Cook until the clams are heated through. Do not boil — it makes the clams rubbery!

Makes 10 servings.

Good Mood analysis

Each serving contains 1 bread; 2 vegetables; 2 very lean proteins; 1 fat; 4 grams dietary fiber.

Spinach-Tofu Dip

I use this instead of sour cream dip all the time. No one can tell the difference — the trick is to use silken tofu. And no one will even know they're eating soy.

16 ounces silken tofu
1 package (1½ ounces) dry onion soup/dip mix
1 package (8 ounces) frozen spinach, thawed, drained, and chopped
1 can (6 ounces) water chestnuts, drained and diced

Combine the tofu and soup mix in a food processor. Whip the mixture until smooth. Add the spinach and process until desired consistency. Fold in the water chestnuts.

Serve with whole-wheat Melba rounds.

Makes 12 servings.

Good Mood analysis

Each serving contains 1½ vegetables; 2 grams dietary fiber.

Smoked-Fish Pâté

This savory pâté can be joined with whole-wheat bread for an easy lunch, or spread on crackers for an elegant appetizer for guests. Talk about versatile fish . . .

1 pound smoked fish (white fish, bluefish, or trout), boned and skinned
⅓ cup reduced-fat mayonnaise
1 tablespoon chopped fresh parsley
2 tablespoons minced onion
½ cup Neufchâtel cheese (light cream cheese)

In a blender, puree all the ingredients until well mixed.

Makes 4 servings.

Good Mood analysis

Each serving contains 4 lean proteins.

English-Muffin Pizzas

This makes a great quick and easy lunch or, cut into triangles, simple hors d'oeuvres (for entertaining). Kids will love it from the first bite.

     2 tablespoons pizza sauce
     1 whole-grain English muffin, split
     2 to 3 tablespoons shredded low-fat mozzarella cheese
     ½ cup chopped veggies such as green pepper, olive, mushrooms
         (optional)

Preheat the oven to 450°F. Spread the pizza sauce onto the muffin halves. Sprinkle with the cheese and veggies. Bake for 10 minutes.

Makes 1 serving.

Good Mood analysis

Each serving contains 1 vegetable (optional); 2 breads; 1 medium-fat protein; 6 grams dietary fiber.

Chocolate Popcorn

Here's a fast snack that I'm sure will become a new favorite in your house. Chocolate makes popcorn a special treat — no matter what age you are. And it elevates popcorn to a super-mood booster.

    1 bag (2.9 ounces) low-fat microwave popcorn
    1 bar (4.5 ounces) bittersweet chocolate, finely chopped
    ½ cup sliced almonds

Pop the popcorn in the microwave according to package instructions. While the popcorn is still hot, toss with the chocolate until the popcorn is evenly coated. Add the almonds and toss again.

Makes 4 servings.

Good Mood analysis

Each serving contains 1 bread; 3 fats; 3 teaspoons added sugar; 6 grams dietary fiber.

Onion Pie

Consider this Good Mood comfort food, but it also doubles as a healthy alternative to quiche.

    1 French bread refrigerator dough (11 ounces)
    8 ounces mushrooms, sliced
    3 large onions, thinly sliced
    2 tablespoons olive oil
    2 cups shredded low-fat Colby and Monterey Jack cheese
    3 eggs, beaten
    salt and pepper, to taste

Spray an 8-inch pie plate with nonstick cooking spray. Roll out the dough and place in the pie plate, cutting off the excess. Bake for 10 minutes according to the package directions, or until it is set but not browned.

Meanwhile, sauté the onions and mushrooms in the olive oil. Drain off **all** the excess liquid. Add the cheese, eggs, salt, and pepper and mix well.

Pour the onion mixture into the pie crust and bake until the center is set and the crust is brown, about 25 minutes.

Makes 6 servings.

Good Mood analysis

Each serving contains 2 breads; 2 vegetables; 3 medium-fat proteins; 1 fat; 3 grams dietary fiber.

Spinach Strudel

If you're going to be on the Good Mood Diet for life, you need to have foods that you can serve to company or just make for yourself and still feel good about. Strudel is a great comfort food and this recipe is beautiful and easy.

½ cup minced shallots
2 tablespoons olive oil
1 package (10 ounces) frozen spinach, thawed and drained
4 ounces feta cheese
4 ounces fat-free cottage cheese
¼ cup chopped fresh parsley
3 eggs, beaten
salt and pepper, to taste
6 sheets frozen phyllo dough (thawed overnight in refrigerator)

Preheat the oven to 350°F.

Sauté the shallots in the olive oil. Set aside until cool. In a mixing bowl, combine the cooled shallots, spinach, feta cheese, cottage cheese, and parsley. Mix in the eggs. Season with salt and pepper and set aside.

Place one sheet of phyllo on parchment paper. Spray the leaf with butter-flavored nonstick cooking spray and cover with a second phyllo leaf. Continue until all 6 leaves are stacked together. Place the spinach mixture along one long side of strudel. Using the parchment as a support, roll strudel into a long cylinder, but don't roll it up with the parchment.

Place the strudel and parchment on a baking sheet with the seam on the bottom. Bake 30 to 40 minutes, or until golden brown.

Makes 12 servings.

Good Mood analysis

Each serving contains 1½ vegetables; 1 very lean protein; 1 fat; 1 gram dietary fiber.

Tuna Noodle Casserole

Taking a traditional favorite and making it healthier is always a plus. If you like a kick to your casserole, use low-fat pepper-jack cheese for half of the cheddar. The nutrition was analyzed using a healthy tuna with 3.5 grams of fat per ounce.

2 tablespoons Smart Balance 67% Buttery Spread
1 cup sliced fresh mushrooms
½ cup diced onion
1 cup frozen peas
2 cans (12 ounces each) fat-free evaporated milk
2 tablespoons flour
8 ounces whole-wheat noodles, cooked
1 can (12 ounces) tuna packed in water, drained and flaked
1½ cups shredded low-fat cheddar cheese
salt and pepper, to taste

Preheat the oven to 350°F.

Melt the spread in a large skillet over medium heat. Add the mushrooms and onion and sauté. Add the peas and evaporated milk. Bring the mixture to a boil. Sprinkle flour over the mixture and stir until mixture thickens, about 3 minutes.

In casserole dish, combine the noodles, tuna, cheese, and sauce; mix well. Bake for 30 minutes.

Makes 6 servings.

Good Mood analysis

Each serving contains 2 breads; 1 vegetable; 5 very lean proteins; 2 fats; 3 grams dietary fiber.

Turkey Meat Loaf

Meat loaf is one of those weekly family rituals that most of us have left behind. This recipe is better than retro; the turkey will lift your mood along with making new and healthier memories of family and friends.

Note on alternative use: Place tablespoons of the turkey mixture into mushroom caps and broil 5 to 10 minutes.

4 slices whole-wheat bread, toasted and torn into pieces
1 pound ground turkey
1 onion, minced
2 eggs
1 small can (3 ounces) tomato paste
1 teaspoon dried basil
½ teaspoon minced garlic
1 small can (6 ounces) diced canned Italian seasoned tomatoes
6 fresh basil leaves, chopped

Preheat the oven to 400°F.

Place the toasted bread in a food processor and blend until crumbed. Add the turkey, onion, eggs, tomato paste, dried basil, and garlic and blend until mixed.

Form a loaf with the meat mixture and place in a baking dish. Cover with the diced tomatoes. Bake the loaf 30 minutes, or until a meat thermometer registers 165°F when inserted in the middle of the loaf. Garnish with fresh chopped basil.

Makes 4 servings.

Good Mood analysis

Each serving contains 1 bread; 2 vegetables; 4 lean proteins; 4 grams dietary fiber.

Fesenjan

Don't be intimidated by the number of ingredients: This classic Persian stew is really simple but has complex flavors that will have family and friends raving.

⅔ cup + ¼ cup dried apricots

1 cup boiling water

¼ cup pomegranate juice

¼ cup tomato paste

¼ cup dried plums, chopped

½ teaspoon ground cinnamon

⅛ teaspoon turmeric

⅛ teaspoon ground cardamom

⅛ teaspoon ground cloves

⅛ teaspoon ground ginger

1 medium onion, chopped

1 tablespoon olive oil

1 pound boneless turkey breast, cubed

½ cup chopped walnuts

3 cups cooked brown rice

Soak ⅔ cup apricots in the boiling water until very soft, 30 minutes. Transfer to a blender and puree. Transfer to a large saucepan. Chop the remaining ¼ cup apricots and add to the puree, along with the pomegranate juice, tomato paste, dried plums, and spices. Bring to a boil and simmer for 15 minutes.

Meanwhile, sauté the onion in the olive oil. Add the turkey and cook until browned and cooked through. Add the turkey mixture and walnuts to the apricot mixture and cook an additional 10 minutes.

Serve over brown rice.

Makes 6 servings.

Good Mood analysis

Each serving contains 1 bread; 2 fruits; 4 very lean proteins; 2 fats; 4 grams dietary fiber.

Pan-Asian Halibut

This recipe has been a family favorite for many years. It is so easy to make and serve, no one will believe that it took you only five minutes to do the preparation. And it makes you *feel so good!*

½ cup aged apple cider vinegar (or regular apple cider)
2 tablespoons tamari or soy sauce
1½ teaspoons toasted sesame oil
2 garlic cloves, minced
1 teaspoon minced fresh ginger (or ½ teaspoon ginger juice)
12 ounces halibut steak
cilantro sprigs, for garnish

In a small glass baking dish, mix together the vinegar, tamari, sesame oil, garlic, and ginger. Add the halibut and turn to coat. Cover and marinate 30 minutes, or up to 4 hours in the refrigerator.

Preheat the oven to 350°F. Bake the halibut in 20 to 25 minutes, until just cooked through. Transfer the fish to a baking sheet and place under the broiler for 3 to 5 minutes, or until browned but not burned. Serve garnished with sprigs of cilantro.

Makes 2 servings.

Good Mood analysis

Each serving contains 5 very lean proteins; 1 fat.

Turkey Braid

This beautiful dish is perfect for entertaining! You can eat healthy, yet have gorgeous and delicious food.

  1½ pounds boneless turkey, cooked and cubed
  1 cup fat-free mayonnaise
  ½ cup chopped walnuts
  ½ cup dried cranberries
  3 tablespoons yellow mustard
  ½ cup shredded low-fat cheese (optional)
  salt and pepper, to taste
  1 can (11 ounces) French bread dough (from the refrigerator case)

Preheat the oven to 375°F.

In a large bowl, combine the turkey, mayonnaise, walnuts, cranberries, mustard, cheese, salt, and pepper.

Unroll the dough and place the filling in the middle third of the dough. Cut the dough flaps into strips, leaving them attached to the middle. Alternate crossing the dough over the turkey salad to form a braid.

Bake 30 to 40 minutes, or until golden brown.

Makes 8 servings.

Good Mood analysis

Each serving contains 2 breads; 4 very lean proteins; 2 fats (cheese included); 2 grams dietary fiber.

Citrus Cobb Salad

We don't usually make elaborate salads for ourselves at home. But you should try this easy recipe — it makes you feel like you're eating at a lovely seaside restaurant.

4 cups spring salad greens
8 ounces cooked shelled shrimp
1 avocado, peeled and diced
1 can black beans, drained and rinsed
2 small roma tomatoes, seeded and julienned
1 can (11 ounces) mandarin oranges, drained
8 black olives, pitted and sliced
1 cup shredded low-fat cheddar cheese
8 fresh asparagus spears, grilled in olive oil and garlic
Citrus Vinaigrette (opposite)

Place greens into four individual bowls. Run a row of shrimp down the center of the greens. Add strips of avocado, beans, tomatoes, orange pieces, olives, cheese, and asparagus. Drizzle the vinaigrette on top.

Makes 4 servings.

Good Mood analysis for the salad with vinaigrette

Each serving contains ½ bread; ⅔ fruit; 3 vegetables; 2 very lean proteins; 1 medium-fat protein; 4 fats; 12 grams dietary fiber.

Citrus Vinaigrette

You might like this dressing enough to make it one of your staples. Feel free to store it in the fridge for a week.

½ cup orange juice
½ cup olive oil
2 tablespoons rice vinegar
1 tablespoon minced parsley
1 teaspoon grated lemon zest
½ teaspoon minced garlic
dash salt and pepper

Combine ingredients in a bottle with lid. Shake until well combined. Let the vinaigrette stand at least 1 hour to blend flavors. Shake before serving.

Mole Poblano Turkey

Olé for mole! What a mood booster, with chocolate and turkey in the same dish. This mole, while flavorful, does not have a lot of heat. If you like spicy hot Mexican food, add 1 to 2 seeded dried chile peppers to the ancho chiles.

½ cup chicken broth, plus more if needed

⅛ dried ancho chile, seeded

½ cup almonds, processed until smooth in the food processor

1 onion, chopped

1 cup drained canned Italian plum tomatoes

½ cup lightly packed seedless raisins

½ cup pumpkin seeds

1 corn tortilla, torn into small pieces

1 teaspoon finely chopped garlic

1 teaspoon salt

1 teaspoon ancho chile powder

½ teaspoon ground cinnamon

½ teaspoon ground cloves

½ teaspoon ground coriander seeds

¼ teaspoon freshly ground black pepper

2 pounds boneless turkey, cubed

½ cup olive oil

3 ounces unsweetened chocolate, chopped

Bring ½ cup broth to a boil. Remove from the heat and add the ancho chile; rehydrate about 30 minutes. In a food processor, combine the rehydrated chiles, almond butter, onion, tomatoes, raisins, pamplan seeds, tortilla, garlic, and spices. Process until smooth.

Transfer to a large saucepan and cook on low for 30 minutes, stirring to prevent burning. Add additional broth for desired consistency.

Meanwhile, in a fry pan, brown the turkey in the olive oil until cooked through.

Add the chocolate to the mole sauce and stir until melted. Add the turkey and cook an additional 5 minutes.

Makes 8 servings.

Good Mood analysis

Each serving contains ½ fruit; 3 vegetables; 5 lean proteins; 2 fats; 8 grams dietary fiber.

Caramelized Brussels Sprouts

While my produce experts at Sosio's stand at Pike Place Market call these "little green balls of death," you'll love this recipe. If you avoid cooked Brussels sprouts because of their sulfurous odor, this recipe eliminates that problem by sautéing them instead of boiling.

    2 tablespoons olive oil
    1 tablespoon minced garlic
    10 ounces Brussels sprouts, cleaned and quartered
    ½ red bell pepper, julienned
    salt and pepper, to taste
    crushed red pepper (optional)

Heat the oil in a nonstick skillet. Add the garlic and sauté until light brown. Add the Brussels sprouts. **Do not stir.** Cook until the bottoms of the sprouts begin to caramelize or brown.

Stir and reposition Brussels sprouts so nonbrowned sides are down. Add the bell pepper and continue cooking until the pepper is soft. Stir to prevent burning. Season with salt, pepper, and crushed red pepper.

Makes 4 servings.

Good Mood analysis

Each serving contains 1 vegetable; 1 fat; 2 grams dietary fiber.

Braised Broccoli Rabe with Currants and Pine Nuts

12 ounces broccoli rabe

1 small onion, minced

2 teaspoons minced fresh ginger

2 tablespoons olive oil

½ cup dried currants

½ cup pine nuts

⅓ cup vegetable stock

2 tablespoons balsamic vinegar

2 teaspoons Splenda

salt and pepper, to taste

Preheat the oven to 350°F.

In an oven-proof casserole, sauté the broccoli rabe, onion, and ginger in the oil. Add the currants, pine nuts, stock, vinegar, and Splenda.

Cover and bake 10 minutes. Season with salt and pepper.

Makes 4 servings.

Good Mood analysis

Each serving contains 1 fruit; 1 vegetable; 3 fats; 2 grams dietary fiber.

Holiday Cranberry Sauce

In our house, this sauce makes regular appearances. It is just too delicious and healthy to save for once or twice a year.

12 ounces fresh cranberries
¼ cup water
Splenda, to taste

Boil the cranberries in pot with water until they pop and burst. Remove from the heat and mix in Splenda to taste.

Makes 6 servings.

Good Mood analysis

Each serving contains 1 vegetable; 2 grams dietary fiber.

French Toast

This classic recipe needs little explanation, just loved ones ready to eat.

2 eggs, lightly beaten
½ cup low-fat milk
½ teaspoon vanilla extract
½ teaspoon ground cinnamon
4 slices whole-wheat bread
Maple syrup (optional)

Combine the eggs, milk, vanilla, and cinnamon in a shallow bowl. Dip the bread in the egg mixture and allow to soak about 30 seconds each side.

Lightly spray a large skillet with nonstick cooking spray. In batches if necessary, add the bread and cook, turning once, until nicely browned. Serve with maple syrup, if you like.

Makes 2 servings.

Good Mood analysis

Each serving contains 2 breads; 1 medium-fat protein; 4 grams dietary fiber.

French Cheese Twist

1½ cups fat-free ricotta cheese

¼ cup Splenda

1 egg

1 teaspoon vanilla extract

1 teaspoon ground cinnamon

1 can (11 ounces) French bread dough (from the refrigerator case)

Preheat the oven to 350°F.

In a small bowl, combine the ricotta, Splenda, egg, vanilla, and cinnamon. Set aside. On parchment paper unroll the dough to a rectangle. Spoon the cheese mixture down the center of the dough.

With a knife, slice horizontal 1-inch-thick strips from each side of the dough, but do not cut into the cheese so that the center stays whole. From the top, criss-cross the strips over the cheese, alternating the strips from left to right, like a braid, until you reach the middle. Start at the other end so that the last braid appears in the center. Twist the 4 ends together to form a knot at the center of the loaf.

Bake 30 minutes, or until browned.

Makes 8 servings.

Good Mood analysis

Each serving contains 1⅓ breads; 1 very lean protein.

Cheese Pancakes

Serve these for breakfast, brunch, or even dessert. They're sweet enough that they don't need syrup.

1 cup fat-free ricotta cheese
½ cup whole-wheat flour
½ cup raisins
2 eggs, lightly beaten
1 tablespoon Splenda
1 teaspoon cinnamon
1 teaspoon vanilla extract

In a medium bowl, combine all the ingredients; mix well. Heat a griddle over high heat. Spray with nonstick cooking spray.

In batches, spoon dollops of ⅓ cup batter onto the griddle. Cook until the bottoms have set and begun to brown. Turn and continue cooking until the pancakes are cooked through but not dried out.

Makes 4 servings.

Good Mood analysis

Each serving contains 1 bread; 1 lean protein; 2 grams dietary fiber.

Whole-Wheat Pancakes with Fresh Blueberry Sauce

It's hard to think of a better way to spend a leisurely weekend morning!

2¼ cups whole-wheat flour

2 tablespoons Splenda

1 teaspoon baking powder

½ teaspoon baking soda

½ teaspoon salt

⅔ cup buttermilk

2 large eggs, lightly beaten

1 tablespoon canola oil

Fresh Blueberry Sauce (below)

In a large bowl, combine the whole-wheat flour, Splenda, baking powder, baking soda, and salt. Add the buttermilk, eggs, and canola oil. Stir lightly until dry ingredients have been incorporated. **Do not overstir.**

In batches, spoon dollops of ⅓ cup batter into a nonstick skillet over medium heat. Cook until the bubbles break on the surface, about 3 minutes. Turn and cook on second side until golden brown. Serve with blueberry sauce.

Makes 6 servings.

Good Mood analysis for the pancakes with sauce:

Each serving contains 1 bread; ½ fruit; 1 medium-fat protein; 7 grams dietary protein.

Fresh Blueberry Sauce

2 cups blueberries

1 cup water

2 tablespoons Splenda

1 teaspoon lemon juice

Combine the blueberries, water, Splenda, and lemon juice in a small pan. Bring to a simmer and cook until the berries are soft and begin to burst. Use warm over pancakes or refrigerate and use later.

Flaxseed Muffins

Combine one of these delicious muffins with the Citrus Cobb Salad (page 172), and you've got a winning Good Mood combination.

1 cup dried currants
½ cup all-purpose unbleached flour
½ cup whole-wheat flour
½ cup chopped walnuts
3 tablespoons flaxseed, ground
⅓ cup Splenda
2 tablespoons sugar
1½ teaspoons baking powder
½ teaspoon baking soda
⅛ teaspoon salt
2 large eggs
½ cup carbohydrate-controlled sugar-free yogurt (vanilla or fruit
    flavors are fine)
2 tablespoons canola oil

Preheat the oven to 400°F.

In a medium bowl, combine the currants, flours, walnuts, flaxseed, Splenda, sugar, baking powder, baking soda, and salt. Set aside. In a large bowl, combine the eggs, yogurt, and oil.

Add the dry ingredients to the wet ingredients and mix by hand until the flour is incorporated. Spoon into 12 paper-lined muffin cups. Bake 20 to 25 minutes, until toothpick removes cleanly.

Makes 12 muffins.

Good Mood analysis

Each muffin contains 1 bread; 1½ fats; 3 grams dietary fiber.

Breakfast Tortilla

This classic Southwestern treat has become mainstream. This version gives you a great filling breakfast to start out the day.

    1 medium potato, peeled and cubed

    1 tablespoon olive oil

    1 small onion, finely chopped

    1 teaspoon paprika

    2 eggs, beaten

    ½ cup shredded pepper-Jack cheese

    2 (6-inch) corn tortillas

    ⅓ cup salsa

In a small bowl, microwave the potato on high, or potato, setting for 3 minutes. Heat the oil in a medium skillet and sauté the potato and onion until the onion softens. Add the paprika and continue cooking until the potato begins to brown and is cooked through. Add the egg and cheese and cook, stirring often to prevent burning and to allow even cooking, until eggs have set.

Place the tortillas in the microwave, covered with a damp cloth, and microwave on high 45 seconds, until warmed.

Place half the egg mixture on each tortilla. Top with the salsa and roll up.

Makes 2 servings.

Good Mood analysis

Each serving contains 2 breads; 2 medium-fat proteins; 3 fats; 4 grams dietary fiber.

Chocolate Soufflés

It's nice to have a truly decadent treat for those special occasions. For the most special touch, use individual custard cups.

2½ tablespoons unsalted butter

3 ounces dark chocolate

2 large eggs, separated, plus 2 large egg whites, at room temperature

1 tablespoon sugar

1 tablespoon Splenda, plus more if desired

2 teaspoons vanilla extract

1 cup raspberries

Preheat the oven to 350°F. Spray four 4-ounce custard cups with nonstick cooking spray.

Microwave the butter and chocolate together on row until melted. Cool to room temperature.

In a large bowl, beat the 4 egg whites to soft-peak stage; add the sugar and Splenda and beat until incorporated. In a medium bowl, beat the 2 yolks and the chocolate mixture. Add the vanilla. Fold the chocolate mixture into the egg whites.

Spoon into the prepared custard cups; bake 12 to 15 minutes until the outsides are done but the centers are still soft.

While the soufflés are baking, puree ⅔ cup of the raspberries in a blender; strain to remove the seeds. Add 1 to 2 teaspoons Splenda if you prefer this sweeter.

To serve, drizzle the sauce over the soufflés and garnish with the remaining whole raspberries.

Makes 4 servings.

Good Mood analysis

Each serving contains ½ fruit; 1 medium-fat protein; 2 fats; 2 teaspoons added sugar; 4 grams dietary fiber.

Chocolate Pecan Clouds

Like all meringue cookies, it's best to make these on a day that is not humid. When they have completely cooled you can remove them from the parchment paper. Sometimes you need to turn them upside down to let the bottoms dry.

    3 large egg whites, at room temperature
    1 cup Splenda
    1 teaspoon vinegar
    ½ teaspoon salt
    4 tablespoons natural cocoa powder
    1 cup chopped pecans
    1 tablespoon ground cinnamon

Preheat the oven to 275°F.

In a large bowl, beat the egg whites until foamy. Add the Splenda, vinegar, salt, and 2 tablespoons cocoa. Continue beating until the whites are at sharp peak stage. Fold in the pecans.

By one heaping tablespoon, spoon or pipe the egg white mixture onto a parchment paper–covered cookie sheet. Bake 30 minutes. Turn oven to lowest setting and bake 20 minutes more. Dust with the remaining cocoa and the cinnamon.

Makes about 36 cookies.

Good Mood analysis

2 cookies contain: 1 fat; 1 gram dietary fiber.

Chocolate-Cranberry-Pumpkin Muffin Tops

Everyone knows the best part of the muffin is the top. This great snack or dessert allows you a great muffin without wasting anything. And you will stay in Good Mood range.

½ cup whole-wheat flour

½ cup all-purpose unbleached flour

⅓ cup Splenda

½ cup dried cranberries

½ cup chopped walnuts

4 ounces bittersweet chocolate, chopped

2 tablespoons sugar

½ teaspoon baking powder

½ teaspoon baking soda

⅛ teaspoon salt

2 large eggs, lightly beaten

½ cup canned pumpkin

½ cup carbohydrate-controlled sugar-free vanilla cream yogurt

2 teaspoons almond extract

Preheat the oven to 400°F.

In a medium bowl, combine the flours, Splenda, cranberries, walnuts, chocolate, sugar, baking powder, baking soda, and salt. In a large bowl, combine the eggs, pumpkin, yogurt, and extract. Add the dry ingredients to the wet and mix by hand until the dry ingredients are incorporated. **Do not overmix!**

Spoon the batter into 12 equal mounds on a parchment paper–covered baking sheet. Bake about 15 minutes, until toothpick removes cleanly.

Makes 12 muffin tops.

Good Mood analysis

Each muffin top contains: 1½ breads; 1½ fats; 3 grams dietary fiber.

Brownies

No one should have to live without brownies! That's no way to stay in a Good Mood. Don't use commercial plum butter puree — it usually has added sugar.

1 cup Homemade Plum Butter Puree (opposite)

4 large eggs

8 ounces bittersweet chocolate, melted and cooled

¼ cup Smart Balance 67% Buttery Spread

2 tablespoons vanilla extract

2 cups all-purpose unbleached flour

2 cups Splenda

¼ cup natural cocoa powder

1 tablespoon baking powder

½ teaspoon salt

Preheat the oven to 350°F. Spray an 8-inch square baking pan with nonstick cooking spray.

In a large bowl, combine the puree, eggs, chocolate, spread, and vanilla. In a medium bowl, combine the flour, Splenda, cocoa, baking powder, and salt. Add the dry ingredients to the wet and mix to combine.

Pour the batter into the prepared pan. Bake 30 to 40 minutes, or until a toothpick inserted in the center comes out clean. **Do not overbake.**

Makes 16 brownies.

Good Mood analysis

Each brownie contains 2 breads; 2 fats; 3 grams dietary fiber.

Homemade Plum Butter Puree

2 cups dried plums (prunes)
½ cup water

In a small pan, combine the plums and water and heat on low until the plums are soft, about 30 minutes.

In a blender, puree the plums and water until smooth.

Chocolate Shells with Berries

OK, forget about the guilt! It doesn't belong here. Just enjoy these! You might even find bittersweet or semi-sweet chocolate dessert cups at a gourmet store or your supermarket around holiday time.

   3 ounces bittersweet chocolate
   1½ cups carbohydrate-controlled sugar-free vanilla yogurt
   1½ cups blueberries (or other berries)
   fresh mint sprigs

Microwave the chocolate on low. Coat 6 chocolate cup molds with the chocolate or coat 6 disposable tinfoil cupcake liners. Refrigerate until hardened. Unmold the chocolate cups carefully!

To serve, spoon the yogurt into the cups, top with the blueberries, and garnish with the fresh mint.

Makes 6 servings.

Good Mood analysis

Each serving contains ½ milk; ½ fruit; 1 fat; 2 grams dietary fiber.

Stuffed Apricots

16 dried apricots

16 unsalted roasted whole almonds

2 ounces bittersweet chocolate, chopped

½ cup finely chopped almonds

With the point of a sharp knife, make a small slit into each apricot and insert 1 almond.

Microwave the chocolate on low until melted and smooth. Dip each apricot on the cut side into the chocolate and then the chopped nuts. Place on parchment until the chocolate hardens.

Makes 8 servings.

Good Mood analysis

2 stuffed apricots contain 1 fruit; 2 fats; 3 grams dietary fiber.

Vanilla Bean Custard

If you don't like vanilla bean (it will make dots in your vanilla custard), omit the beans and double the vanilla extract.

2 vanilla beans
1 quart 2% milk
4 large eggs, beaten
⅓ cup sugar
⅓ cup Splenda
½ teaspoon vanilla extract
½ teaspoon ground cinnamon
½ teaspoon ground nutmeg
½ teaspoon salt
1 pint raspberries

Slice the vanilla beans in half and scrape the seeds into the milk then drop the pods in too. In a small pan over medium heat, heat the milk until just before it begins to simmer. Remove from the heat and discard the pods. Let cool.

Preheat the oven to 350°F.

When the milk is cooled, stir in the eggs, sugar, Splenda, vanilla, cinnamon, nutmeg, and salt. Pour into 8 custard cups.

Place the cups in a 9x11-inch pan. Fill the pan halfway with water. Carefully transfer the pan to the oven and bake 45 minutes, until golden brown. Let cool. To serve, top with raspberries.

Makes 8 servings.

Good Mood analysis

Each serving contains ½ milk; ½ very lean protein; 1 fat; 2 teaspoons added sugar.

The Original Good Mood Smoothie

Once you taste this smoothie you'll think that being too busy to sit down and eat is almost worth it. It works great as a periodic meal replacer or a muscle-building snack.

If your whey protein supplement is sweetened, you don't need to add any additional sweetener. If your supplement is plain, then you'll need to add about 1 packet of Splenda.

> 1 cup fat-free milk
> ½ medium banana
> 14 grams protein from isolated whey protein powder
> 1 tablespoon natural peanut butter
> 1 tablespoon natural cocoa powder (non-dutched)
> 1 rounded teaspoon Omega-3 Brain Booster powdered supplement
> 4 to 6 ice cubes

Combine all the ingredients in a blender and blend until smooth, about 1 minute.

Makes 1 serving.

Good Mood analysis

Each serving contains 1 milk; 1 fruit; 3 very lean proteins; 2 fats; 5 grams dietary fiber.

Blackberry Bliss

This pick-me-up is sweet but with a zing!

  1 pint fresh blackberries
  2 teaspoons Splenda
  1 teaspoon pureed fresh ginger
  8 ounces sparkling water (I use Pellegrino)

Juice the blackberries in a juicer; make sure you scrape all the juice from the pour spout, as the juice is thick. In a bowl, combine the juice, Splenda, and ginger; mix thoroughly. Add the sparkling water. Divide the drink between 2 glasses and serve.

Makes 2 servings.

Good Mood analysis:

Each serving contains 1 fruit; 7 grams dietary fiber.

Mango Mambo

Try this smoothie for the next special occasion. It is perfect for a birthday party.

1 mango, peeled and seeded
1 cup fresh-squeezed orange juice (from 3 to 4 oranges)
2 teaspoons Splenda
1 teaspoon almond extract
4 ounces sparkling water (I use Pellegrino)
crushed ice orange peel (optional)

Juice the mango in a juicer; make sure you scrape all the juice from the pour spout, as the juice is thick! In a large bowl, combine the mango juice, orange juice, Splenda, almond extract, and water. Pour over crushed ice in 4 glasses and serve with orange peel twists, if you like.

Makes 4 servings.

Good Mood analysis

Each serving contains 1 fruit; 1 gram dietary fiber.

Renew

What you have been waiting for . . . the anti-aging cocktail in a smoothie glass. And featured on the book cover, no less.

   1 pint fresh red currants
   1 large lemon, juiced (save the peel to make a lemon twist)
   2 tablespoons Splenda
   16 ounces sparkling water (I use Pellegrino)
   crushed ice

Stem the currants. Put through juicer; make sure you scrape all the juice from the pour spout, as the juice is thick! In a large bowl, combine the lemon juice, Splenda, and water. Pour over crushed ice in 2 glasses and serve with lemon peel twists.

Makes 2 servings.

Good Mood analysis

Each serving contains 1 fruit; 5 grams dietary fiber.

Viva

This smoothie is extremely refreshing and packs an energy boost that is hard to match.

    2 cups boiling water
    ¼ cup loose green tea leaves
    1 teaspoon minced fresh lemongrass
    2 cups ice
    2 tablespoons Splenda

In a bowl, pour the boiling water over the tea and lemongrass; allow to steep for 15 to 20 minutes. Strain the tea into a pitcher filled with the ice. Stir in the Splenda. Refrigerate overnight.

Makes 2 servings.

Good Mood analysis

A "free" Good Mood food with no worries.

Metropolitan

This lovely drink will bring to mind a Cosmo, but it will make you feel much better! Try it at your next party or gathering with friends.

    1 red grapefruit, juiced (about ¼ cup)
    ½ lemon, juiced
    ¼ cup sparkling water
    2 tablespoons pomegranate juice
    crushed ice

Combine the grapefruit juice, lemon juice, water, and pomegranate juice. Pour over crushed ice in 2 glasses.

Makes 2 servings.

Good Mood analysis

Each serving contains 1 fruit and a huge serving of fun.

Appendix A

GOOD MOOD FOOD GROUPS

Food Groups	Description	Serving Size
Fluids		
Other Fluids	Water, sugar-free soft drinks, etc.	1 cup (8 ounces)
Wine	Red wine may have some health benefits over white	5 ounces
Vegetables (nonstarchy)		
Carotene-Rich	Carrots, dark leafy greens, tomatoes, yellow squash	1 cup raw, ½ cup cooked
Brassica Family	Broccoli, cauliflower, cabbage, Chinese cabbage, Brussels sprouts, cooked	
Allium Family	Onions, garlic, shallots, chives	
Fruit		
Citrus	Grapefruit	½ large or ½ cup sections
	Orange, lemon, lime	1 small
	Tangerines	2 small

Food Groups	Description	Serving Size
Berries	Blackberries, blueberries	¾ cup
	Raspberries	1 cup
	Strawberries	1¼ cup whole berries
Other	Apple	1 small
	Apple, dried	4 rings
	Applesauce, unsweetened	½ cup
	Apricots, fresh	4 whole
	Apricots, dried	8 halves
	Apricots, canned	½ cup
	Banana	1 small
	Cantaloupe	⅓ small or 1 cup cubes
	Cherries, sweet, fresh	12
	Dates	3
	Figs, fresh	2 medium
	Figs, dried	1
	Grapes	17 small
	Honeydew melon	1 slice or 1 cup cubes
	Kiwi	1
	Mango	½ or ½ cup cubes
	Nectarine	1 small
	Orange	1 small
	Papaya	½ or 1 cup cubes
	Peach	1 medium
	Peaches, canned	½ cup
	Pear	1 medium
	Pears, canned	½ cup
	Pineapple, fresh	¾ cup
	Pineapple, canned	½ cup
	Plums	2 small
	Plums, dried (prunes)	3
	Raisins	2 tablespoons
	Watermelon	1 slice or 1¼ cup cubes
Juice	Apple juice, cider; grapefruit, orange, pineapple juice	½ cup

Food Groups	Description	Serving Size
	Cranberry juice cocktail, reduced-calorie	1 cup
	Fruit juice blends, 100% juice; grape, prune juice	⅓ cup

Bread, Cereal, Starchy Vegetables

Food Groups	Description	Serving Size
Bread	Whole-grain bread	1 slice or 1 ounce
	Whole-grain bun	½
	Bagel, English muffin, pita	½
	Whole-grain pancake or waffle, 4-inch diameter	1
	Tortilla, corn or flour, 6-inch diameter	1
Cereal	Cooked cereal	½ cup
	Shredded wheat	½ cup
	Kashi cereal	1 cup
Rice	Brown rice (preferable) or white rice, cooked	½ cup
Pasta	Pasta and couscous, cooked	½ cup
Vegetables	Corn, cooked	½ cup
	Corn on the cob	1 small cob
	Peas, green	½ cup
	Plantain	½ cup
	Potato, medium, boiled or mashed	½ or ½ cup
	Potato, small, baked with skin	1
	Squash, winter (acorn, butternut, pumpkin)	1 cup
	Yam, sweet potato	½ cup
Other	Crackers, whole-wheat	2 to 5
	Matzo	¾ ounce
	Popcorn, air-popped	3 cups
	Pretzels	¾ ounce
	Rice cakes, 4-inch diameter	2
	Tortilla chips, baked	15 to 20

Food Groups	Description	Serving Size
Fat-free and Low-fat Milk and Dairy (0 to 1 percent fat)		
	Milk, buttermilk, fortified soy milk (all count toward total daily fluid intake)	8 ounces (1 cup)
	Yogurt, plain or with non-caloric sweetener	1 cup
	Yogurt, fat-free, flavored, with non-caloric sweetener	1 cup
Very Lean Protein		
Poultry	Skinless, white-meat chicken and turkey, Cornish hen	1 ounce
Seafood	Fresh or frozen cod, flounder, haddock, halibut, trout, lox (smoked salmon), tuna (fresh or canned in water)	1 ounce
	Clams, crab, lobster, scallops, shrimp, imitation shellfish	1 ounce
Game	Skinless duck or pheasant, venison, buffalo, ostrich	1 ounce
Dairy	Cheese with less than 1 gram fat per ounce:	
	Fat-free or low-fat cottage cheese	¼ cup
	Fat-free cheese	1 ounce
Other	Processed sandwich meats with less than 1 gram fat per ounce, such as deli thin, shaved meats, turkey, ham	1 ounce
	Egg whites	2
	Egg substitute, plain	¼ cup

Food Groups	Description	Serving Size
Beans, Legumes (count as 1 very lean protein plus 1 starch)		
	Adzuki, black, garbanzo, pinto, navy, soy, white beans, cooked	½ cup
	Edamame, cooked in shell	½ cup
	Soy nuts	¼ cup
Lean Protein		
Poultry	Skinless dark-meat chicken, turkey, duck	1 ounce
Seafood	Herring (uncreamed or smoked), salmon (fresh or canned), catfish, tuna (canned in oil, drained)	1 ounce
	Oysters	6 medium
	Sardines (canned)	2 medium
Dairy	Cottage cheese (4½ percent fat)	½ cup
	Grated Parmesan	2 tablespoons
	Cheese with less than 3 grams fat per ounce	1 ounce
Beef and Game	USDA Select or Choice beef, trimmed of fat, including round, sirloin, flank steak, tenderloin, roast (rib, chuck, rump), steak (T-bone, porterhouse, cubed), ground round	1 ounce
	Lean veal chop, veal roast	1 ounce
	Rabbit, goose (well-drained of fat)	1 ounce
Pork	Fresh ham; canned, cured or boiled ham; Canadian bacon; pork tenderloin, center loin chop	1 ounce
Lamb	Lamb roast, chop, or leg	1 ounce
Other	Processed sandwich meat with less than 3 grams fat per ounce (turkey pastrami)	1 ounce

Food Groups	Description	Serving Size
Medium-Fat Protein		
Poultry	Chicken (dark meat with skin), ground turkey or chicken, fried chicken (with skin)	1 ounce
Seafood	Any fried fish product	1 ounce
Dairy	Cheese with less than 5 grams fat per ounce:	
	Feta, mozzarella	1 ounce
	Ricotta	¼ cup (2 ounces)
Beef	Most beef products fall into this category (ground beef, meat loaf, corned beef, short ribs, prime grades of meat trimmed of fat such as prime rib)	1 ounce
	Veal cutlet	1 ounce
Pork	Pork top loin, pork chop, Boston butt, pork cutlet	1 ounce
Lamb	Lamb rib roast, ground lamb	1 ounce
Other	Whole egg	1
	Sausage with less than 5 grams fat per ounce	1 ounce
	Tempeh	½ cup
	Tofu	½ cup (4 ounces)
High-fat Protein		
	All regular cheeses, such as American, cheddar, Monterey Jack, Swiss	1 ounce
	Peanut butter	1 tablespoon
Fat		
Oils	Olive, sesame, canola, peanut, corn, safflower, soybean oils	1 teaspoon

Food Groups	Description	Serving Size
Olives	Black olives	8 large
	Green olives, stuffed	10 large
Nuts and Seeds	Almonds, cashews, mixed (50 percent peanuts)	6 nuts
	Peanuts	10 nuts
	Pecans, walnuts	4 halves
	Pumpkin, sesame, sunflower seeds	1 tablespoon
Nut and Seed Butters	Peanut, almond, cashew butter	½ tablespoon
	Tahini or sesame paste	2 teaspoons
Dressings	Mayonnaise, soy-based, regular	1 teaspoon
	Mayonnaise, soy-based, reduced-fat	1 tablespoon
	Salad dressing, regular	1 tablespoon
	Salad dressing, reduced-fat	2 tablespoons
Dairy	Cream, half-and-half	2 tablespoons
	Cream cheese, regular	1 tablespoon
	Cream cheese, reduced-fat	1½ tablespoons
	Sour cream, regular	2 tablespoons
	Sour cream, reduced-fat	3 tablespoons
Other	Avocado, medium	⅛ (2 tablespoons)

Fish and Seafood (high in omega-3 fats)

	Salmon, halibut, tuna, mackerel, sardines, cod, black cod, rockfish, flounder, sablefish, anchovies, herring, trout, shrimp, scallops, oysters, clams, crab, lobster	1 ounce

Added Sugar

	Eliminate during first two weeks
	Avoid high fructose corn syrup
	See Appendix C (page 217) for teaspoons of added sugar in packaged foods

Food Groups	Description	Serving Size
Supplements		
	Protein from isolated whey protein powder	14 to 21 grams
	Ground flaxseed	1 to 2 tablespoons

Appendix B

GOOD MOOD LOG

Maintaining a log is documented in research studies as a highly effective way to improve health habits. Keeping track of your Good Mood foods will help you see that your favorite meals and snacks can be part of the plan, and you will be more aware of needing to eat every few hours for best results. These log pages hit the highlights of your Good Mood approach. Plus, it can be fun to monitor how great you feel while losing weight.

What I Ate   (Date:_____)

Breakfast

_____ Bread

_____ Fruit

_____ Milk

_____ Medium-fat protein

_____ Fat

_____ Ounces water

Morning Snack

_____ Milk

_____ Very lean protein

_____ Fruit

Lunch

_____ Bread

_____ Vegetable

_____ Very lean protein

_____ Fat

Afternoon Snack

_____ Fruit

_____ Vegetable

_____ Fat

_____ Very lean protein

Dinner

_____ Bread

_____ Fruit

_____ Vegetable

_____ Lean protein

_____ Very lean protein

_____ Fat

Evening Cocoa

Did you have one? _____

"Instant Good Mood Food" Checklist

Even on the most busy day, log whether you are consuming these super-good-mood foods (circle yes or no) that provide virtually an instant lift:

1 whole egg?	Yes	No
1 tablespoon ground flaxseed?	Yes	No
14 grams protein from whey protein powder (21 grams if you are highly active)?	Yes	No
5 to 6 cups water?	Yes	No

Comments: _____

_____

_____

How I Exercised

What type? _____

How long? _____

Number of steps on pedometer: _____

Comments: _____

_____

_____

Good Mood Bottom Line

How did I feel today? _____

_____

_____

_____

_____

_____

_____

_____

_____

_____

_____

_____

Appendix C

ADDED SUGAR IN PROCESSED FOODS

These values are calculated using the amounts of sugar known to naturally be in food and then comparing those to the values of sugar listed on the nutrition facts label of packaged foods. For each category, we looked at a range of products based on price and use of natural ingredients.

You can do the same thing by comparing the amount of sugar in a certain product to an unsweetened version of the product. Note that **4 grams sugar = 1 teaspoon.**

You might find products that have more or less sugar than listed here; these are just average amounts. So make sure to check all the packaged products that you buy.

Check out this list: You'll be surprised at how many foods have added sugar that you never suspected. Always look for the brands with less added sugar.

Food	Serving Size	Teaspoons of Added Sugar
Apple sauce, unsweetened	½ cup	0
Apple sauce, sweetened	½ cup	2
BBQ sauce	2 tablespoons	3 to 4
Beans, baked	½ cup	0 to 4
Bread	1 slice	0 to 1

Food	Serving Size	Teaspoons of Added Sugar
Cereal, cooked, unsweetened	1 cup	0
Cereal, cooked, sweetened	1 cup	1 to 4
Cereal, dry, unsweetened	1 cup	0
Cereal, dry, sweetened	1 cup	1 to 5 (or more)
Cereal bars	1 bar	2 to 5
Chocolate syrup	2 tablespoons	4 to 5
Corn syrup	2 tablespoons	3 to 4
Crackers	1 ounce	0 to 3
Cranberries, dried, unsweetened	¼ cup	0
Cranberries, dried, sweetened	¼ cup	3
Croutons	1 ounce	<1
Domino D 'Lite*	1 teaspoon	1
Equal Sugar Lite*	1 teaspoon	1
Fruit, canned, in juice	½ cup	0
Fruit, canned, in light syrup	½ cup	1
Fruit, canned, in heavy syrup	½ cup	2
Honey	1 tablespoon	4
Hot chocolate, sweetened	1 cup	3
Jam, jelly, fruit spread	1 tablespoon	0 to 3
Juice, apple, unsweetened	1 cup	0
Juice, apple, sweetened	1 cup	1 to 3
Juice, cranberry	1 cup	½ to 6
Ketchup	2 tablespoons	2
Ketchup, low-carb	1 tablespoon	0
Maple syrup, artificial	¼ cup	10
Maple syrup, artificial, lite	¼ cup	6
Maple syrup, artificial, sugar-free	¼ cup	11 grams sugar alcohol
Maple syrup, natural	¼ cup	12
Mayonnaise	2 tablespoons	0
Milk, white	1 cup	0
Milk, flavored	1 cup	4

Food	Serving Size	Teaspoons of Added Sugar
Molasses	1 tablespoon	3 to 4
Mustard, yellow	1 teaspoon	0
Mustard, flavored	1 teaspoon	½
Pancake mix	⅓ cup mix	0 to 2
Peanut butter, natural	2 tablespoons	0
Peanut butter, conventional	2 tablespoons	1
Pickle relish	1 tablespoon	1
Pickles	1 ounce	0 to 2
Pie filling	½ cup	4
Raisins	¼ cup	0
Rice, plain	half cup	0
Rice, flavored	½ cup	1
Salad dressing	2 tablespoons	½ to 2
Salsa	2 tablespoons	0 to 1
Soft drink, regular	12 ounces	10
Soft drink, diet	12 ounces	0 to 2
Soup, canned	1 cup	0 to 1
Splenda	1 teaspoon	0
Splenda Baking*	1 teaspoon	1
Sports drinks	1 cup	3 to 6
Sundae topping	2 tablespoons	5 to 6
Sundae topping, sugar-free	2 tablespoons	19 to 24 grams sugar alcohol
Tomato or pasta sauce	½ cup	1 to 2
Yogurt	½ cup	0 to 8

Based on manufacturer's data and authors' calculations
*sweeter than regular sugar, so you need less.

CHAPTER NOTES

Chapter 1: Feel-Great Foods

1. The federal daily recommended limit for cholesterol is 300 milligrams for the healthy adult. Most nutritionists agree with that amount, and the Good Mood Diet daily menu plans presented in chapter 3 average 300 milligrams per day. I have figured your morning egg into the equation.

   What especially keeps you in alignment with cholesterol guidelines is following the lean protein and dairy servings and skipping the fried and processed foods. Saturated fats in fatty meats and whole milk (or 2 percent) and trans fats that form in fried and processed foods cause the body to produce its own cholesterol. Eggs are low in saturated fat — provided you don't, say, fry them in butter or cover them with a cream sauce.

   A couple of other points: the American Heart Association estimates one large, whole egg contains 213 milligrams of cholesterol, or 71 percent of the healthy max. Extra-large and jumbo eggs check in at 93 percent of the max.

   Mother Earth News, a magazine dedicated to the return of "real food" to our dining tables, tested the cholesterol content of free-range chicken flocks and found that those eggs (from heritage breeds) had about half the cholesterol of conventional eggs. As an added bonus, the eggs contained up to twice as much vitamin E, up to six times more beta carotene (which helps produce vitamin A in the body), and four times more omega-3 essential fatty acids compared to the U.S. Department of Agriculture standard. The sample size is admittedly small but still turned heads.

   One important caveat: if you have coronary heart disease, diabetes, high LDL cholesterol, or other cardiovascular disease, your doctor might peg your daily cholesterol limit as less than 200 milligrams. Choose one small or medium egg, with 157 or 187 milligrams of cholesterol respectively, and note that the Good Mood menus recommend soy substitutes to help you with the daily limit.

On the brain food front, University of North Carolina public health researcher Steven Zeisel has published a number of studies that make a case for getting more of the brain chemical choline into our daily meals, especially for women (*Journal of the American College of Nutrition,* Vol. 23, No. 90006, 621S–626S, 2004). The richest sources of choline include beef and chicken liver and eggs. I say pass on the liver and go for the daily egg.

2. Canadian researcher Terry Graham, who runs the human biology and nutrition department at the University of Guelph in Ontario, has conducted and published several recent lab studies showing that caffeine increases insulin resistance, at least for a few hours.

Quick refresher: insulin resistance is not good. It can lead to type 2 diabetes. Graham's findings seem to represent a reason to reevaluate your daily coffee pattern. Most experts agree that cutting back on your afternoon or evening consumption is a wise step. By doing that you give the body — specifically the central nervous system — a chance to recalibrate its insulin response overnight.

"The increasing effect of coffee on insulin resistance is acute in the here and now," says Graham. "We know it lasts for a few hours."

Here's a paradox that Graham has described. While his lab studies show a temporary acute spike in insulin resistance, long-term epidemiological research shows that the risk of type 2 diabetes goes down significantly among heavy coffee drinkers. Just the opposite of what the Guelph studies indicate. "Welcome to science," says Graham, chuckling.

How you make your coffee changes its impact. The French press method, for example, is known to produce more caffeine than other techniques.

When you drink coffee also matters. The full effect of caffeine reaches the bloodstream about 45 to 60 minutes after you drink coffee, tea, or caffeinated soda. Graham reveals himself as being in alignment with the Good Mood approach to morning coffees and lattes. "I quit coffee a few years ago," says Graham. "I observe a lot of the negative effects in our research studies. But I started drinking it again because I like it and I have the distinct advantage of knowing exactly how it affects my insulin resistance." Graham averages about two to three cups per day, which he says fits just fine in his fitness program. "My only rule is to finish my day's coffee by lunchtime," says Graham. "That's because I like to sleep at night."

3. There are several good sources to study up on mercury content in canned tuna. One of the best reports, entitled "Mercury Rising," was published by a *Chicago Tribune* investigative team in late 2005, prompting formal promises by the federal government to more closely regulate the type of tuna put into cans. The *Tribune* revealed that the U.S. tuna industry is using a potentially high-mercury tuna species, yellowfin, in about 15 percent of the 1.2 billion

cans of light tuna sold annually. Most of these cans are not labeled yellowfin, making it impossible for consumers to know which cans might be high in mercury.

Other good sources of information about mercury in seafood include the Washington, DC–based nonprofit Environmental Working Group (www. ewg.org) and fishing-savvy Washington state's Mercury Education Project (www.mercurymess.org).

4. I highly recommend checking out the work of Gregory S. Berns, an associate professor of psychiatry and behavioral sciences at Emory University in Atlanta, especially his fascinating book, *Satisfaction: The Science of Finding True Fulfillment* (Henry Holt & Co., 2005). He is a pioneer in connecting how the brain responds when we feel satisfied versus happy versus content and much more. His Web site has lots of citations if you want to dig into the science: www.ccnl.emory.edu/greg/.

A landmark study related to brain imaging and food was performed by researchers from the National Institute of Diabetes and Kidney Diseases and published in the June 2002 issue of the *American Journal of Clinical Nutrition*. It was the first to show that men and women respond to food differently, at least in terms of PET (positron emission topography) images showing the brain's blood flow.

The scans revealed many similarities between the men's and women's brains during hunger and satiation, but there were differences such as, when hungry, men had more activity than women did in the paralimbic region of the brain, an area involved in processing emotion. When sated, women had more activity than men did in the occipital cortex, the seat of vision, and men had more activity than women did in an area of the prefrontal cortex, associated with feelings of satisfaction.

What that all means will be a subject of research studies and debate for, oh, at least a good decade, probably more.

5. One example: a joint study by Netherlands and Yale University researchers (*American Journal of Clinical Nutrition*, Vol. 75, No. 6, 1051–1056, June 2002) showed that whey increases the brain's ratio of plasma tryptophan, which leads to greater serotonin production and boosts mood. Better yet, whey enhances cognitive performance during times of stress. You are more alert and less frazzled.

Plus, whey protein is connected with promoting weight loss, especially if you couple your midmorning smoothie with daily exercise (best case is to drink the shake after exercise). An October 2005 study published in the journal *Nutrition* (Vol. 21, No. 10, 1052–1058) suggested that whey protein can play an important role in discouraging hepatic fatty acid synthesis. Translation: you accumulate less body fat because the whey stimulates muscle tissue to burn more fat during exercise.

6. I won't do this to you often, but here is a compact bibliography of scientific citations that link food and mood, especially our feelings of being down or depressed. I think it is important to show that science has weighed in

early and often on the subject. These studies focus on whether dieting —
effectively limiting carbohydrates — affects mood and depression:

Anderson, I. M., Parry-Billings, M., Newsholme, E. A., Fairburn, C. G., and
Cowen, P. J. (1990). Dieting reduces plasma tryptophan and alters brain
5-HT function in women. *Psychological Medicine,* 20, 785–791.

Goodwin, G. M., Cowen, P. J., Fairburn, C. G., Parry-Billings, M., Calder,
P. C., and Newsholme, E. A. (1990). Plasma concentrations of tryptophan
and dieting. *British Medical Journal,* 300, 1499–1500.

Greiwe, J. S., Holloszy, J. O., and Semenkovich, C. F. (2000). Exercise induces
lipoprotein lipase and GLUT-4 protein in muscle independent of adrener-
gic-receptor signaling. *Journal of Applied Physiology,* 89, 176–181.

Schweiger, U., Laessle, R., Kittl, S., Dickhaut, B., Schweiger, M., and Pirke,
K. M. (1986). Macronutrient intake, [plasma large neutral amino acids] and
mood during weight-reducing diets. *Journal of Neural Transmission,* 67,
77–86.

Wolfe, B. E., Metzger, E. D., and Stollar, C. (1997). The effects of dieting on
plasma tryptophan concentration and food intake in healthy women. *Physiology and Behaviour,* 61, 537–541.

Wurtman, R. J., and Wurtman, J. J. (1995). Brain serotonin, carbohydrate-
craving, obesity and depression. *Obesity Research,* 3, 477S–480S.

7. Experimental studies suggest that marine fatty acids have an antitumor effect
on prostate tumor cells. A 2003 study published in the journal *Cancer Epi-
demiology Biomarkers & Prevention* (Vol. 12, 64–67, January 2003) followed
47,882 men participating in the Health Professionals Follow-up Study. Eating
fish more than three times per week was associated with a reduced risk of
prostate cancer and especially discouraged the spread of cancer outside the
prostate.

8. Joseph Hibbeln, a psychiatrist and biochemist from the National Institutes of
Health, is someone who shows up as a coauthor in many studies related to the
mood-enhancing properties of "good" fats such as cold-water fish and flax.
Hibbeln says he believes the increasing incidence of depression may be due to
diets containing the wrong sorts of fats.

Here's his take: the brain is made up mostly of fat, and it is argued that the
consumption of omega-3 unsaturated fats, rather than omega-6 fats, can reduce the incidence of depression. Convenience-driven changes in the typical
American diet have reduced omega-3 fats and increased omega-6 fats (corn
oil, other vegetable oils, and processed foods). Hibbeln says this could well be
leading to sharp increases in depressive illnesses. He says eating more fish,
flaxseed, and walnuts could be a better solution to depression than taking antidepressants. I wholeheartedly agree.

Chapter 2: Feel-Bad Foods (It's a Short List)

1. Purdue University nutrition researcher Richard Mattes has performed a
number of studies related to satiety. He has consistently found that people feel

more full from a handful of nuts compared to other snacks that might seem healthier (rice cakes), heavier (pickles are used in some experiments), or less fatty (chestnuts, which are higher in carbs than most nuts). While these other choices satisfied appetite for about a half hour on average, nuts worked much longer in staving off hunger.

2. The researchers are Dr. James Rohrer, a family medicine practitioner at the Mayo Clinic, and Dr. David L. Katz, director of the Prevention Research Center at Yale University School of Medicine. The article was first posted December 4, 2005, at www.biomedcentral.com/bmcpublichealth, one of the growing number of Internet research journals.

   If you are looking to study up on your alcohol habits — maybe during your two-week Good Mood hiatus? — then Carl Erickson is your man. He is director of the Addiction Science Research and Education Center at the University of Texas in Austin. Erickson has developed an extensive and annotated Web site related to 300 alcohol facts (www.utexas.edu/research/asrec). Among other useful information, he has posted clear definitions of "moderate" and "social" drinking.

   Moderate use of alcohol, he writes, has been defined by the Department of Agriculture (and other sources) as one to two drinks per day — one drink for women, two drinks for men. He points out that moderate drinking is associated with reduced risk of heart disease (and possibly with preventing diabetes and strokes) but that the "mechanism of the protective effect is unknown."

   Erickson defines "social use" of alcohol as "an occasional drink or two in the company of friends: a glass of champagne at a wedding, a cold beer after a softball game, or a glass of fine wine with a meal. . . . Contrary to popular belief, social drinking does not kill brain cells, nor does it adversely affect any major body organ," he writes.

   Another eye-opener: women clearly are more affected by alcohol. Erickson explains that women break down alcohol more slowly than men because there is a smaller amount of alcohol-metabolizing enzyme (alcohol dehydrogenase) in women's stomachs.

3. Recent studies investigating tea and health have linked tea drinking with positive health effects on cardiovascular diseases, cancer, insulin activity, bone mineral density, arthritis, and even cataracts (Yang, C. S. and Landau, J. M. [2000]. "Effects of tea consumption on nutrition and health," *Journal of Nutrition,* 130, 2409–2412).

   The thermogenic effect of tea has generally been attributed to its caffeine content. Now researchers are finding that it may not be the caffeine alone but the interaction of other important compounds called catechin-polyphenols in the tea with caffeine that produces the greatest thermogenic effect, along with the added bonus of increased fat burning. Green tea is a particularly potent source of epigallocatechin gallate, one of the most bioactive catechin-polyphenols.

   How about this news-you-can-use entry for what you should add to your tea: a group of researchers in Beltsville, Maryland, investigated the influence of catechins on insulin activity (Nagao, T., Komine, Y., Soga, S., Otsuca, K., Meguro, S., W Eatanabe, H., Hase, T., Tamaka, Y., Tokimitsu, I. [2002]. "Long-term intake of tea catechins reduces body fat in men," *International Journal of Obesity and Related Metabolic Disorders,* 26, S158). Reduced insulin sensitivity is one of the areas being investigated as a possible precursor or consequence of obesity.

Enhancing insulin sensitivity may help overweight individuals lose weight or manage body composition. In laboratory cell culture studies, tea was shown to increase insulin activity more than 15 times. Black, green, and oolong teas but not herbal teas were shown to increase insulin activity. The addition of lemon to the tea did not affect the insulin-potentiating activity, but the addition of one teaspoon of 2 percent milk per cup decreased the insulin-potentiating activity by one-third. When about one-quarter of a cup of milk was added, the insulin-potentiating activity nearly disappeared. Non-dairy creamers and soy milk also decreased the activity.

The amount of tea you need to consume isn't really clear. It appears to be somewhere between two and six cups daily. If you are caffeine sensitive, you might want to start with the lower dose, and definitely don't drink the tea in the evening before bed. Cheers!

Chapter 3: The Good Mood Plan and Fourteen Days of Menus

1. See previous note for the green tea background.

Chapter 4: The Good Mood Kitchen

1. Stress means different things to each of us. How diet and stress interact is, well, a whole other book. But one of the landmark findings about stress is that it commonly equates to feeling a lack of control in situations. The classic study looked at British civil workers at various levels on the organizational chart. You might assume that supervisors, especially middle managers both answering to bosses and being responsible for the production of underlings, would be most stressed out. Not so. The most stressed individuals were the lowest-level workers, who basically felt no control in any part of their jobs.

2. I can tell you from professional experience that keeping a food diary is a powerful tool for clients. Three detailed days (two "normal" days and one weekend day) is more than enough to enlighten people and motivate change.

    Data from the National Weight Loss Registry confirms the value of keeping food journals. And there are other examples of how writing it down reinforces good habits.

    Consider the University of Michigan's DrinkWise alcohol moderation program. Researchers and counselors require participants to keep a regular diary of their alcohol habits — and they say it is one of two key factors in downsizing alcohol intake (the other is abstaining for two weeks at the start of the program — sound familiar?). The counselors have consistently found that participants change their ways simply by documenting what they do, especially noting what they don't want to do in the future.

It is a documented fact that research subjects who drink moderately to heavily underestimate their alcohol consumption in self-reports. British researchers discovered that using a diary doesn't stop the underestimating but does result in more truth about how rapidly drinks are consumed (this speed dictates how fast or slowly alcohol gets into the bloodstream) and how many times in a week or month someone becomes intoxicated.

3. This outcome is frequently assumed, but a 2002 University of Washington study of Seattle-area kids put the pesticide pass-through effect to the test (Curl, C.L., Fenske, R.A., and Elgethun, K. "Organophosphorus pesticide exposure of urban and suburban pre-school children with organic and conventional diets," *Environmental Health Perspectives,* published online, October 13, 2002). It found that kids who eat conventionally grown produce have higher chemical blood levels related to pesticides.

That study bookends with a 2006 finding that confirms organic diets will significantly lower children's exposure to widely used pesticides *(Environmental Health Perspectives,* Vol. 114, Number 2, February 2006). It is the first study to conduct a longitudinal analysis of children's pesticide exposure and represents a joint effort between the University of Washington's Richard A. Fenske from the 2002 study and researchers at Emory University and federal Centers for Disease Control and Prevention in Atlanta.

4. This debate will go on for a good long while. One concept that is indisputable is "food miles." No one can deny that shipping produce across the country (mostly from California) or from other continents (South America, New Zealand) cannot provide the same freshness as picking up local produce at neighborhood farmers' markets. That freshness equates with flavor.

5. The most important recent book out there on organic and whole foods is Michael Pollan's *Omnivore's Dilemma: A Natural History of Four Meals* (Penguin Press, 2006). He covers Brix scores and much more in his delightful narrative style (featured often in the pages of the *New York Times Magazine).* He traces four different meals — industrial, industrial organic (a scary and inevitable category), grass-fed (also called "beyond organic") and hunter-gatherer — to in part track how much processed food — especially corn derivatives — we eat in this country. Hint: it's not pretty.

6. See note 3 in Chapter 1.

Chapter 5: The Good Mood Traveler

1. It probably won't surprise you that this study was partly funded by a dairy industry trade association. But the findings make sense to me. I have long reminded my athlete-clients to not forget chocolate milk as a quick, convenient, and effective pick-me-up after a practice or game. The citation is *International Journal of Sport Nutrition and Exercise Metabolism* (2006; 16: 78–91).

The small study was designed for nine cyclists to ride to exhaustion, then take a four-hour break before riding a second session to exhaustion. During the rest period, the cyclists were provided one of three drinks: low-fat chocolate milk, a traditional fluid replacement sports drink, or a carbohydrate replacement sports drink.

The researchers found that the cyclists who drank chocolate milk during the rest period were able to bike nearly twice as long before reaching exhaustion as those who consumed the carbohydrate replacement drink, and as long as those who consumed the fluid replacement drink.

"Chocolate milk contains an optimal carbohydrate-to-protein ratio, which is critical for helping refuel tired muscles after strenuous exercise and can enable athletes to exercise at a high intensity during subsequent workouts," says coauthor Joel M. Stager, professor of kinesiology at Indiana University.

2. One of the first widely reported celery studies was the 1992 experiment at the University of Chicago Medical Center. In an animal lab, researchers injected a chemical extract from celery into rats. The result was that the celery extract, a substance called 3-n-butyl phthalide, worked to smooth the muscles that line the blood vessels, in turn lowering blood pressure by an average of 12 to 14 percent. The comparable daily dose of 3-n-butyl phthalide for adults is equal to four stalks of celery a day.

In China, the research about celery as a blood pressure remedy is long-standing. Same goes for the folklore medicine factor. In fact, one of the University of Chicago researchers was inspired to do the study because his father refused to eat less salt as a way to decrease blood pressure. Instead, the father ate a quarter-pound of celery each day for a week. Seven days later, his blood pressure had dropped from an elevated level of 158 over 96 to a normal level of 118 over 82.

Chapter 6: Good Mood X-Factors: Exercise and Rest

1. Honestly, I remember this statistic from my undergraduate psychology classes. Ergonomics researchers have updated break time to about every 20 minutes for at least getting up to stretch and move out of the computer hunch position. If you are interested in deeper research, do a Web search for Australian researcher Wendy Macdonald at the Centre for Ergonomics and Human Factors at La Trobe University in Australia. Here are two citations:
W. Macdonald (2003). "Workload and Work Stress," Chapter 6 in *Work Stress: Studies of the Context, Content and Outcomes of Stress. A Book of Readings.* New York: Baywood Publishing.
W. Macdonald (2003). The impact of job demands and workload on stress and fatigue. *Australian Psychologist*, 38, 2, 102–117.

2. University of Tennessee exercise scientist Dixie Thompson published the first study specifically identifying the number of steps necessary for healthy weight (measured here as body mass index, or BMI). Her primary intent was to develop a walking formula for midlife women.

"Those who walked less had more total fat, and more centrally located fat," Thompson writes. Here's the citation: Thompson, D. Relationship Between Accumulated Walking and Body Composition in Middle-Aged Women, *Medicine & Science in Sports & Exercise,* May 2004, 911–914.

3. See previous note.

4. Here is a link to Bartholomew and his study: www.utexas.edu/opa/news/2006/01/education17.html. The citation is "Effects of acute exercise on mood and well-being in patients with major depressive disorder," *Medicine & Science in Sports & Exercise,* 37(12):2032–2037, December 2005.

5. There are studies that make the case for stretching after your muscles get warm and others that contend stretching either before or after a workout does nothing to prevent injury. What seems indisputable is that stretching will improve your flexibility. And most every practitioner agrees that warming up the muscles, even for five minutes of aerobic activity, before stretching is best.

   "When the temperature of muscles is higher than normal, stiffness decreases and extensibility increases," says Michael J. Alter, author of *Sport Stretch* (Human Kinetics). Dr. Lyle J. Micheli, an orthopedic surgeon at Harvard Medical School and past president of the American College of Sports Medicine, says that stretching for five minutes after exercise prevents muscles from tightening too quickly. He suggests athletes go through an abbreviated version of the stretches performed before an activity.

Chapter 7: Good Mood Momentum: Keeping It Going

1. Variety in our foods and tastes reduces the brain's perception of satiety or feeling full. Researchers Hollie A. Raynor and Leonard H. Epstein at the University of Buffalo discovered that people overeat when they are in a situation when they can taste different foods (holiday dinners and Sunday brunch buffets come to mind). The field of research is called "sensory-specific satiety." Raynor and Epstein performed a meta-analysis of 58 studies, finding, interestingly, similar satiety patterns in both humans and animals. ("Dietary Variety, Energy Regulation, and Obesity," *Psychological Bulletin,* Vol. 127, No. 3, 2001.)

2. See note 1 for Chapter 1.

3. See note 2 for Chapter 4.

ACKNOWLEDGMENTS

The Good Mood Diet has been a work in progress for twenty-five years. Counseling athletes who need to enhance not only their physical energy but also their mental stamina, mood, and focus, I delved into the neuroscience literature to begin to understand the biochemistry of the brain. I wanted to learn about the influence of food on emotion, cognitive function, and brain health. If I ever went back to school, I would study neuroscience.

I am convinced that by furthering our knowledge of the brain and the continuum of the mind-body connection, we will begin to solve the enigma of the obesity epidemic. I want to acknowledge and thank two great scientists for explaining their work in a way that I could understand and apply to my own field. In that spirit, I thank Dr. Eric Kandel and Dr. Gregory Berns for their inspirational works and books on the science of memory, learning, emotion, and mind.

To Bob Condor, my coauthor and professional acquaintance for more than a decade, thank you for sharing my vision, reporting on the Good Mood Diet (originally called the Daylight Diet), and giving your insightful journalistic touch to the Good Mood Diet story.

To Jill Cohen, former publisher, and Karen Murgolo, editorial director, of Springboard Press, thanks for your confidence in my work. I knew when I met you both that everything felt right. And thank you to Jamie Raab, publisher of Warner Books, who now oversees Springboard Press. We also appreciate the dedication and hard work of copy editors extraordinaire Peggy Freudenthal and Deri Reed.

To Roger Oglesby, editor and publisher of the *Seattle Post-Intelligencer,* thank you for referring my diet idea to your editors and health columnist.

To my agent, Al Zuckerman, thank you for encouraging me to pursue my passion. Your advice has given me the confidence to step out of my comfort zone. To Claire Zuckerman, your sharp editorial pencil and your clear support of the program were crucial to the early phases of this journey, and greatly appreciated.

To Karen Friedman-Kester, MS, RD, LD, we have shared a friendship and professional partnership for many years. Thank you for your culinary expertise and recipes that make the Good Mood Diet appetizing and delicious.

The success of the Good Mood Diet Clubs (AKA Daylight Diet) in Seattle began with the members of the *Seattle Post-Intelligencer* group, and then continued and expanded with the support of Karla Anderson and her expertise in movement and exercise. Karla, thank you for being such an enthusiastic cheerleader and exercise guide.

To all the participants of the Good Mood Diet Clubs and to the clients that I have worked with during the past several years, your comments and input into the development of the program have been invaluable. I couldn't have done it without you, and your experiences have been my inspiration to write the book.

To my family: Jeff, you taught me that excellence is a worthwhile goal. Whether at work or at play, if you're going to do something, give it all you've got. Thank you for pursuing life with me with passion for the past twenty-five years. To Danielle and Ilana, you have taught me so much, you keep me in the moment and you make me laugh. Thank you for your patience and your unconditional love. To Mom, you are the original Good Mood Dieter. Thanks for believing in me. To Chuck, Judy, Maddy, Stephen, and Amy, you have listened to my stories, encouraged me to step out on a limb, and ski down a slope that I would never have tried on my own. Surrounded by all of you, who wouldn't be in a good mood?

—DR. SUSAN M. KLEINER

When I left my position as sports editor of the *Chicago Tribune* in early 1994, I was excited for the new challenge of starting a health and fitness beat at the *Tribune.* I left my figurative front-row seat with some lasting impressions from watching athletes up close — especially Michael Jordan and his three-peat champion Chicago Bulls teammates. One standout lesson was how much training and nutrition could improve both your physical and mental performance. I figured it was time to help the newspaper's readers achieve the same results.

One of the first sources I called on the new beat was Dr. Susan M. Kleiner.

She was a sports nutritionist with a top-notch reputation among Seattle athletes and various Olympians. By phone, I realized Susan's personal supply of energy was right up there with her elite clients. She was quoted in my first story (about whether we really needed to drink eight glasses of water) and appeared in numerous stories and columns of mine since then. Now that I live in the Seattle area, we've even had the pleasure to eat a Good Mood lunch now and then.

To Susan, I say thanks for devoting the hours and effort necessary to work with the *Seattle Post-Intelligencer* test group — and for asking me to be part of the book project. And thanks for your never-fail dose of encouragement throughout the process.

To the Daylight Dieters, Jennifer Lail, Paula Burke, Benito Cervantes, Patrick D'Amelio, Felicity Mansanarez, and Sharon Lee Hamilton, thanks for your openness and spirited participation. You were chosen from more than a hundred and fifty candidates and each of you was a terrific choice.

To Karen Murgolo, our editor and the editorial director of Springboard Press, we appreciate your guidance and wisdom every step of the way. To Matthew Ballast and Cassandra McCann, thanks for taking on the publicity and marketing efforts to get out the Good Mood Diet message. Peggy Freudenthal and Deri Reed were invaluable as copy editors. And thanks to Jim Schiff for pulling together many production elements.

To my editors at the *Seattle Post-Intelligencer,* Roger Oglesby, David McCumber, Chris Berenger, Stephanie Reid-Simons, Bob Schenet, and John Engstrom, I never take for granted the privilege of column space in the *P-I.* Your professionalism and friendship are stellar. Also, a huge thanks to photographer Joshua Trijillo.

I would like to thank some friends and editors at the *Chicago Tribune,* who believed in me and smoothed my transition from sports to the health beat: Jim Warren, Denise Joyce, Ross Werland, Nancy Watkins, Geoff Brown, Ann Marie Lipinski, and, not least, Rick Kogan, who assigned me that first article about water and handed me column space a couple of months later. I am always feeling good about that group.

To my family — now there's where Good Mood flows the most for me. To my wife and forever soulmate, Mary, who still fuels my each and every day. To our children, Arthur and Lana, who see the world through wide eyes, earnest minds, and open hearts, I learn something new from each of you every day. Plus, even better, I am reminded that the present is what we are guaranteed, so let's enjoy it and savor it.

—BOB CONDOR

INDEX

afternoon snack. *See also* Good Mood
   Diet menus; snacks
   Good Mood Template, 56
air-popped popcorn, 11, 47, 123
alcohol
   combining and, 44
   depression and, 138
   as Feel-Bad Food, 11, 40
   food diary and, 226–27n. 2
   moderate use of, 42, 43, 60–61, 225n. 2
   momentum builders and, 150, 151
   sleep and, 139
   social use of, 50, 225n. 2
   timing of, 44
   two-week abstinence from, 12, 42, 43,
      44, 60
allergies, 109–10, 146
almonds, 17, 33, 39, 146
alpha-linolenic acid (ALA), 35, 107, 115,
   116
Alter, Michael J., 229n. 5
American College of Sports Medicine,
   132–33, 135, 137–38
American Heart Association, 134, 221n. 1
anchovies, 23, 35
appetite. *See also* hunger
   alcohol consumption and, 43
   hot cocoa and, 5
   satiation of, 39

appetizer recipes
   Smoked-Fish Pâté, 158
   Spinach-Tofu Dip, 157
appetizers, in restaurants, 126
apples, 122
apricots, Stuffed Apricots, 195
Asian food, 100

bacon, 17, 45
baked potatoes, 99
bathroom scales, 144
beans, 209
bean soups, 99
Behlke, Linda, 24, 117
Bencetic, Sherry, 4, 9
Berns, Gregory S., 137, 223n. 4
berries, 79, 102, 206
Black Bean Salsa Soup, 154
Blackberry Bliss, 199
blenders, 97
blood sugar, 30, 33
blueberries, as Feel-Great Food, 11
blueberry recipes, Fresh Blueberry Sauce,
   183
body-fat percentage, lowering of, 27
brain
   chemical changes in, 4, 8, 16
   eggs as beneficial to, 17, 146, 222n. 1
   emotional outcome of choices and, 148